# WITHDRAWN
## UTSA LIBRARIES

# IICAPS

# IICAPS

A Home-Based

Psychiatric Treatment for

Children and Adolescents

Joseph L. Woolston, M.D.
Jean A. Adnopoz, M.P.H.
and Steven J. Berkowitz, M.D.

Yale University Press   New Haven & London

Set in Adobe Garamond and Stone Sans types by
Integrated Book Technology, Troy, New York.
Printed in the United States of America.

*Library of Congress Cataloging-in-Publication Data*

Woolston, Joseph L.
    IICAPS : a home-based psychiatric treatment for children and adolescents /
Joseph L. Woolston, Jean A. Adnopoz, and Steven J. Berkowitz.
        p. ; cm.
    Includes bibliographical references and index.
    ISBN 978-0-300-11249-8 (cloth : alk. paper)

    1. IICAPS. I. Adnopoz, Jean. II. Berkowitz, Steven J. (Steven Jay) III. Title.
[DNLM: 1. IICAPS.    2. Mental Health Services—Connecticut.
3. Adolescent—Connecticut.    4. Child—Connecticut.    5. Family Therapy—
Connecticut.    6. Home Care Services—Connecticut.    7. Mental Disorders—
therapy—Connecticut.    8. Models, Organizational—Connecticut. WM 30
W916i 2007]
    RJ502.4W66 2007
    362.198'92009746—dc22                                            2007017890

A catalogue record for this book is available from the British Library.

The paper in this book meets the guidelines for permanence and durability of
the Committee on Production Guidelines for Book Longevity of the Council
on Library Resources.

10  9  8  7  6  5  4  3  2  1

# Contents

# Acknowledgments

The Intensive In-Home Child and Adolescent Psychiatric Service (IICAPS) at Yale University is a team model. IICAPS interventions are co-constructions of parents, clinicians, and supervisors. The development of the IICAPS model was a parallel co-construction of the authors and the initial program coordinators and staff. We are particularly indebted to Cecilia Rowland, Ed.D., Virginia DeVarennes, LCSW, and Elizabeth Rodriguez, Ph.D., whose supervisory skills and knowledge of the client families were indispensable. We are grateful for the expertise and good humor of Kathleen Balestracci, Ph.D., our primary data analyst. We express our heartfelt thanks to Kristin Holdt, LCSW, and Cecilia Singh, Ph.D., for their ability to manage the essential tasks of training, data collection, monitoring, consultation, and credentialing. We are deeply appreciative of the sustained efforts of Timothy Odaynik, Leena Kennedy, Anne Santello, and Brian Rebeschi of the Child Study Center and Frank Gregory, Ph.D., and Robert Plant, Ph.D., of the Department of Children and Families. Mark Schaefer, Ph.D., of the Department of Social Services, and Robin Weersing, Ph.D., of the Child Study Center, have helped to guide us on our journey toward becoming an evidence-based treatment. In addition, we wish to acknowledge the children and families served by IICAPS programs throughout the state that have joined with us and enabled us to learn together.

# Abbreviations

CASSP: Child and Adolescent Service System Program

DCF: Department of Children and Families

DSS: Department of Social Services

EBT: evidence-based treatment

IICAPS: Intensive In-Home Child and Adolescent Psychiatric Service

MAOA: Monoamine oxidase A

MST: multisystemic therapy

PTSD: Post-Traumatic Stress Disorder

SED: serious emotional disturbance

YICAPS: Yale Intensive In-Home Child and Adolescent Psychiatric Service

# Chapter 1 Introduction

The severity of the current crisis in children's mental health has led to increased scrutiny of existing treatments and resources (Satcher, 2000; State of Connecticut, 2000). Considerable attention has been focused on the implementation of new models of care that demonstrate the potential both to improve outcomes for children with serious psychiatric disorders and to relieve the distressed condition of the mental health system. This volume addresses the service system issues confronting contemporary mental health providers and planners, describes in detail a model of home-based psychiatric care that is proving to be effective in reducing reliance on in-patient and other institution-based services, and outlines some of the remaining unresolved challenges to providing effective home and community-based care.

The model, the Intensive In-Home Child and Adolescent Psychiatric Service (IICAPS), is central to the contention that in-home care is a viable and sound treatment option for children with serious psychiatric disorders. IICAPS was initially developed by the authors in 1996 to assist in the transition of children with serious emotional disturbance (SED) from psychiatric hospital to home or to prevent unnecessary placement in more restrictive facilities. Initially implemented in New Haven, Connecticut, IICAPS is currently being replicated in 13 sites across the state. A structured, manualized intervention, IICAPS relies on training, supervision, and specific tools and procedures to support staff to adhere consistently to the model. Adherence is believed to be central to the delivery of IICAPS services. Rooted in the integration of clinical knowledge, theory, and research, the IICAPS treatment approach has its origins in the history of mental health services in the United States. The IICAPS model offers a replicable response to contemporary demands for evidence-based, child-focused, family-driven community services.

## MENTAL HEALTH SERVICES FOR CHILDREN: THE CURRENT CRISIS

During the past decade, the mental health systems caring for children and adolescents have been increasingly overwhelmed by the rapid rise in the number of children who are affected by psychiatric disorders severe enough to compromise their ability to remain safely in their homes and communities. Many of these children have required repeated treatments in hospital settings, experienced frequent visits to hospital emergency departments, or been placed in foster care or residential treatment facilities (Satcher, 2000; State of Connecticut, 2000; President's New Freedom Commission on Mental Health, 2003). While the cost of treating these children has continued to escalate, neither the quality nor quantity of services available to them has shown marked improvement. In some documented cases, the quality of the care available has been found to have significant and wide-ranging deficiencies (*New York Times,* September 1, 2003). In 19 states where such data are tracked, including California, Connecticut, Florida, Pennsylvania, Minnesota, and Texas, public child welfare and juvenile justice systems have been asked by families to assume custody of their mentally ill children because they cannot bear the cost of providing care. This is a deplorable practice that further stresses already inadequate systems and places children at increased risk of suffering the additional consequences of removal from their families and communities (ibid.; President's New Freedom Commission on Mental Health, 2003).

The gridlock resulting from overstrained mental health systems, the high costs of care, the profit-seeking behavior of managed care entities, and the immediate needs of the estimated four million children with SED has precipitated a crisis in the children's mental health system. A report presented to the Connecticut General Assembly (Connecticut Department of Social Services, 2000) found that although some children with SED required and received the highest level of care, many others, who could have been treated in their homes and communities with appropriate resources, were being maintained unnecessarily in hospitals or institutions because of the lack of community-based resources available to assist their families to support them.

Between July and December 1999, 55 percent of the children in the custody of Connecticut's Department of Children and Families (DCF) were in acute care psychiatric hospitals and medically ready for discharge to less-intensive community settings, but there was nowhere for them to go (Connecticut Department of Social Services, 2000). Similarly, residential treatment facilities were also at or near capacity, yet many of the children in residential treatment no longer needed this level of care. These conditions reflected the insufficient number of community-based services available to maintain children at risk of in-patient treatment in their own homes or to support their successful and timely return from more restrictive care to their families and communities. Although this report was specific to conditions in Connecticut, the situation that it describes is ubiquitous. Mental health systems throughout the United States that purport to serve children and adolescents have been paralyzed by gridlock and constrained by their failure to develop innovative, developmentally sound, and financially viable alternative solutions.

The prevalence of diagnosable mental health disorders in children in the United States presents a significant challenge to the service system. An estimated one-fifth of all American children are affected by some type of mental health problem. A subset of children receiving mental health services, estimated between 5 and 9 percent, suffers from severe emotional disturbance and associated functional impairment. Although not all children with mental health disorders enter the service system, those with impaired functioning require strenuous and sustained intervention. The cost of providing services to these children is significant. Although estimates vary, researchers using 9 percent of the total dollars expended on mental health services across the life cycle as a relative measure conclude that more than $7 billion is being spent annually for services for children and adolescents (Friedman, Kutash, and Duchnowski, 1996; Marsh and Fristad, 2002). The soundness of this investment is called into question in a report published by Barbara Burns and Robert Friedman that found that in-patient and residential treatment centers, the least researched and most costly interventions, consumed three-fourths of the treatment dollars (Burns, Hoagwood, and Mrazek, 1999). These findings were replicated in a report prepared for the Connecticut Department of

Social Services in 2000 by the Child Health and Development Institute of Connecticut. This report found that 70 percent of all state behavioral health dollars were spent on psychiatric hospitalization and residential treatment for 19 percent of the children receiving services paid for by Medicaid.

The magnitude of the problem assumes even greater proportions when consideration is given to the fact that many children, particularly those in the child welfare system who remain in their homes or live with relatives, are in need of mental health care but never receive it (Burns et al., 2004). Given these conditions, it is folly to believe that solely adding hospital beds and expanding residential treatment facilities will break the treatment logjam and improve the system of care.

The report of the Surgeon General of the United States on Children's Mental Health (Satcher, 2000), recognizing the failure of the mental health system to address the multiple needs of children with serious disorders, concluded that the types of problems associated with the treatment of these children were most likely to be remediated through multisystemic interventions that encouraged families and providers to work together collaboratively. Although evaluative research on the effectiveness of multisystemic approaches to the treatment of serious emotional disturbances in children and adolescents was still in its infancy, the report called for the development of integrated systems of care, a philosophy already accepted as the consensus approach (Lyons and Rogers, 2004). When confronted with the inability of existing services to meet the complex and wide-ranging needs of children and families, mental health planners turned attention to the creation of systems of care that were grounded in theories of child development, social ecology, and systems building. These models recognized that functional improvement for the child and positive outcomes for the family would result from including not only the child but also his family, his school, and the others with whom he interacted regularly in the treatment approach (Stroul and Friedman, 1996).

For more than three decades mental health planners, policy makers, and practitioners have demonstrated sustained interest in the systems of care concept. The principles central to systems of care, developed by a consensus of mental health professionals, have been widely accepted. These principles, which hold that services should be community or neighborhood based, culturally responsive, holistic, individualized, integrated, and strength based, are commonly used to inform the development of new programs and services for children with SED and have had widespread influence on professional practice and training. System of care theory views families as full partners in the work of treatment. Respect, cooperation, and collaboration between family members and providers are considered essential elements of effective intervention (Meyers, Kaufman, and Goldman, 1999). It is possible to trace the widespread acceptance of these principles and their influence on resource development through the history of children's mental health services in the United States.

## SYSTEMS-LEVEL INTERVENTION:
## TOP-DOWN CHANGE

For decades the distress and dysfunction of children with serious emotional disorders have challenged the resources of parents, teachers, and community services (Joint Commission on the Mental Health of Children, 1969; President's Commission on Mental Health, 1978; Saxe et al., 1987). In response, public- and private-sector institutions have funded large-scale initiatives committed to community-based collaborations and system building. These collaborations have been expected to promote the development of healthy, productive children and to reduce dependence on programs and facilities that sever children's ties to their biologic families. The initial effort to create a mental health system for children in the United States can be traced to the adoption of the Community Mental Health Centers Amendment in 1970 (P.L. 91-211), which established a special authority for the provision of services for children in free-standing mental health clinics or in newly created mental health centers. The lack of financial resources hampered the legislative intent. Over time the community mental health centers, which were designed to meet the behavioral health needs of both adults and children, were relieved of their obligation to provide discrete children's services. In 1978 the Carter administration proposed the Children and Youth Mental Health Services Systems Initiative, an attempt by the federal government to support the development of community-based systems of care for children with serious emotional disturbances. Once again, the inadequacy of fiscal resources led to a failed effort; the services created were insufficient to meet the demand. The only administration-supported program initiative to survive was the Indian Health Service, which was able to find the funding necessary to involve communities in the tasks of identifying children in need of services and creating systematic responses to their needs. Nonetheless, within three years the entire initiative disappeared.

In 1980, two years after the report of the President's Commission on Mental Health, Congress passed the Mental Health Systems Act, which once again recommended the development of community-based services for children and adolescents with serious emotional disturbances. However, in 1981 under the new Reagan administration the legislation was repealed, though not without having served a useful purpose. The aims of the legislation were not lost to some legislators and policy makers. An important but usually overlooked aspect of these early initiatives was the failure to recognize that children's developmental issues do not fit neatly into the discrete domains usually addressed by governmental agencies or private provider organizations. Psychologically and behaviorally troubled children and youths are not only served by the mental health system, but they also populate the child welfare, juvenile justice, and education systems. When disturbed and disturbing youths are prevented from receiving services from one system, they may find themselves involved with an alternate system that labels them differently to ensure that they qualify for its services. In some instances entry into one system may increase the child's vulnerability for the problems that are addressed in another system. For example, although referrals for protective services may result in access to resources that may provide real benefits to a child, the risks associated with the intervention may also adversely affect the child's psychological functioning. In fact, the current crisis in mental health underscores the interrelatedness between the multiple systems in which children and families function. Resolving the crisis depends, at least in part, on the persistent development of programs and institutional alliances that recognize that integration across systems and across all functional domains is essential for effective treatment. The majority of youths that are appropriate for one system (for example, mental health) may also be appropriate for other systems (for example, child welfare or juvenile justice). Therefore, it is not surprising that some important legislative remedies for children with mental health problems have emerged from child welfare legislation.

Addressing this point, the Adoption Assistance and Child Welfare Act of 1980 (P.L. 96-272) recognized and endorsed the developmental need of children to remain with their families of origin as long as their safety was not seriously compromised. P.L. 96-272 required states to "prevent the unnecessary separation of children from families by identifying family problems, assisting families to resolve them and preventing family breakup." Although the act made permanence a central goal for all children entering the child welfare system (Wells and Tracy, 1996), policies that address the most appropriate means of assuring permanency for vulnerable children continue to evolve to this day.

The Adoption Assistance and Child Welfare Act was not specific to children diagnosed with psychiatric disorders; rather it was directed toward children reported to child welfare and protective service agencies as abused or neglected. Interestingly, a study by Snyder and McCollum (1999) found that many children in the protective service system were symptomatic for mental health disorders and likely to benefit from treatment, particularly home-based family therapy. However, they also found that few therapists were trained to provide treatment in settings other than traditional outpatient clinics and residential facilities. In addition to expanded services, new training programs and increased attention to clinical supervision would be necessary to meet the challenge of changing treatment venues for children and adolescents with SED from restrictive, out-of-home settings and examining rooms to their homes and communities. It would be years before these issues were addressed robustly.

In 1984 the National Institute of Mental Health (NIMH) initiated the Child and Adolescent Service System Program (CASSP). CASSP was to become one of the most influential of all federal attempts to encourage and support the development of integrated, collaborative systems of care for children with SED. CASSP principles, adopted from system-of-care concepts, underscored the central role to be played by parents as partners and decision makers in all aspects of their children's care, broadened the array of services from traditional individually oriented treatment to include more eclectic approaches to behavioral change, and advocated cultural competence and flexibility. CASSP was designed to achieve four primary goals: (1) the creation of interagency collaborations within each state to address the complex, cross-disciplinary needs of children with SED and their families; (2) increased capacity of state mental health agencies to provide appropriate services for children with SED; (3) expansion of parental involvement in making decisions related to the care and treatment of their SED children; and (4) the development of community-based, advocacy-oriented, multidisciplinary planning processes (Solnit et al., 1997).

CASSP resonated with the findings of advocates like Jane Knitzer, who in a landmark study published in 1982 documented the failure of public mental health agencies to identify and treat the mental health needs of children in the child welfare system. Knitzer and other advocates pressed for fresh approaches to children and adolescents lost in mental health systems that did not fully understand their individual needs or possess the capacity to respond to them (Behar, 1985, 1986; Bickman, 1996). The CASSP strategy supported parental empowerment, multidisciplinary planning, and collaboration among providers and service programs. CASSP principles provided a strong contrast to the more common public agency response to children with SED, a response that relied upon the use of residential institutions and foster-care systems as primary interveners and treaters. However, while CASSP encouraged all the states to apply for federal funding to support systems change initiatives, CASSP dollars could be used only for planning and for reorganization of state mental health service delivery systems. States were prohibited from using CASSP funding to develop new clinical services.

In 1990 the Robert Wood Johnson Foundation provided the first phase of funding needed to expand the availability of services required by the fledgling systems of care as they were developing and to assess the effectiveness of the CASSP approach. The Mental Health Services Program for Youth (MHSPY) created by the foundation enabled 11 states committed to CASSP principles to reform and expand their systems of care for SED children and adolescents. The cornerstone of the CASSP approach was the assumption that coordinated, cross-disciplinary case planning, management, advocacy, and clinical services in which parents are involved as partners would result in functional improvements for children and restoration of their impaired capacities. Other multisite initiatives such as Safe Start, an Office of Justice, Juvenile Delinquency Prevention (OJJDP) program, focused on building multisystemic collaborations for children age 6 and under exposed to violence and trauma, and the Annie E. Casey Child Welfare Program have followed in the footsteps of MHSPY. However, the complexities inherent in these attempts to weave together and address simultaneously both individual needs of children and families and larger systemic issues have made evaluators cautious in drawing comparisons or inferences. In a landmark study of the Fort Bragg continuum of care for children and adolescents, Leonard Bickman et al. (2000) found that children who received mental health treatment in a coordinated system of care did no better than comparison children. Others have found that the skills and core competencies of the mental health professionals providing care may be as integral to the ability of systems of care to demonstrate improvement in the outcomes for children and families as public policy, service mix, and funding sources (Meyers, Kaufman, and Goldman, 1999).

### FOCUSED SYSTEMS CHANGE: FOSTER CARE

Reliance on the foster-care system as an effective intervention for children whose parents were unable to meet their needs undoubtedly created more problems for these children than it cured. The problems resulting from disrupted relationships and educational and geographic discontinuities had a profound influence on development and led to severe impairments of attachment (Bernstein, 2002). Reflecting awareness of the detrimental effects of removing children from familiar settings, the Adoption Assistance and Safe Families Act of 1997, one of the most important pieces of legislation of the past decade, included provisions for financial incentives to states to discourage foster-care drift and to ensure stability, safety, and permanence for high-risk children, who were often without long-term plans. Though not specifically developed as mental health legislation, the act reflected the facts that during the past decade, several pronounced and disturbing trends had emerged concerning children involved in the foster-care system.

Over this period the age of children in out-of-home care had decreased; one-quarter of all children entering the foster-care system in the five largest states were under the age of six (Berrick et al., 1997). Additionally, although children entering foster care were more likely to be victims of trauma and to suffer from chronic medical conditions and mental health disorders (Brereton, 2000), they often failed to receive the health care necessary to mitigate these problems while they were in care (U.S. General Accounting Office, 1995, as cited in Brereton, 2000). Children placed in foster care were also likely to experience more than one placement. For example, the average number of placements for children in Connecticut who entered the foster-care system in 1995 was 3.5 (Martin, 1995). Data released in 1998 showed that 66 percent of children who were placed outside their homes were eventually reunited with a family member. However, these family members were unlikely to have received any services during the time their children were in placement, nor were they given any assistance in preparing for the child's return (Adnopoz and Ezepchick, 2003). Most disturbingly, the care that was available was often fragmented and inconsistent, since social and medical histories were often left behind as children moved from place to place. As a result, their new caregivers were often uninformed about other areas of the child's life and unprepared to meet behavioral or medical problems as they arose. All these issues raised serious questions about the efficacy of foster care as a treatment option for high-risk children from multiproblem families. Consideration of these issues led to legislation designed to encourage states to develop more effective ways of both meeting the mental health needs of children and families and reducing the potential for damage that could result from placement in a flawed foster-care system.

At the same time that concern was raised about removing children from familiar environments and exposing them to the possible problems of institutional or foster placements, many states were faced by additional issues of great concern: a shortage of institutional beds and an inadequate supply of licensed foster homes in which children could be placed. The combined weight of these factors increased the interest in and support of home- and community-based, child-centered, family-focused interventions as important alternatives for children for whom out-of-home placement might otherwise be seriously considered. Traditional outpatient mental health resources, such as office- or clinic-based treatment, had proved to be a poor fit for work with poorly organized, multiproblem families in which children and parents suffer from multiple, competing problems, including serious mental health disorders. Many of these problems are reactive and cannot be relieved without simultaneous interventions leading to concurrent changes in the environment (Adnopoz, 2005).

## INTERVENTIONS THAT SERVE THE CHILD
## AND FAMILY IN THE HOME

Home- and community-based services had their origins in the nineteenth century when friendly visitors representing charitable organizations called on families to determine their needs and to work with them to increase their self-sufficiency. In the early years of the twentieth century many of these methods were adopted by social workers who recognized the advantages of entering and observing the family's environment firsthand and mobilizing natural, community-based networks (Wells, 1995; Woodford, 1999). It is not surprising that the benefits of working directly in homes of children and their family continue to be robust. When clinicians enter the diagnostically rich, textured, and highly personal environment of each home, they step directly into the family's individual ecology. By making use of their observational skills, clinicians are able to piece together a tapestry of knowledge about the real-world experiences of the child and family that not only facilitates treatment, but is also unavailable to those who see the family exclusively in traditional examining rooms (Adnopoz and Culler, 2000). The process of working in the home enhances the clinician's ability to understand and address the complexity of the dynamic reality that constitutes the everyday world of both children and their parents.

Bringing services to the home also addresses the problems of resistance and access to service that surface regularly with vulnerable populations.

Many families in which children are at high risk for out-of-home care may be difficult to engage and distrustful of the traditional, clinic-based mental health system. Noncompliance with treatment protocols and appointment schedules may occur frequently. As a result children may not receive the level of treatment thought necessary to improve their health and mental health conditions. Importantly, clinicians have found that parents and other family members are more likely to become supportive of and consistently involved in the child's treatment and recovery when appropriate mental health services are delivered directly in the home and community (Adnopoz and Ezepchick, 2003; Woodford, 1999).

In the later decades of the twentieth century advocates such as the Edna McConnell Clark Foundation encouraged and funded states to implement programs that could maintain children in their own homes and communities, promote permanency for the child, reduce the probability of placement outside the home, and prevent the inevitable problems associated with foster-care drift (Nelson, 1988). Homebuilders, an early model of intensive, short-term, home-based intervention for rebellious adolescents developed in Tacoma, Washington, was endorsed by both funders and policy makers. Homebuilders staff worked intensively but briefly with adolescents and their families in their own homes to address the conflicts that threatened the family's cohesion. Outcome data supported the effectiveness of the model and demonstrated significant reduction in the use of out-of-home placements (Kinney and Dittmar, 1995). The belief that maintaining children in their own homes would represent cost savings to taxpayers also supported the popularization of Homebuilders and some of the other so-called family preservation programs that developed on its heels.

A growing body of evidence has supported in-home, family-focused intervention as a necessary component of a comprehensive system of care for children and youths with problems of mental health, substance abuse, and delinquency (Fraser, Hawkins, and Howard, 1988; Kaufman and Kaufman, 1992; Henggeler et al., 1998; Harrison, Boyle, and Farley, 1999). Many of the programs that have been studied offer sustained, relationship-based services that generally address three domains: parent, parent-child, and child functioning (Heinicke and Ponce, 1999). Their success has enabled in-home intervention and treatment to emerge as an effective means of engaging difficult-to-reach families and preparing them to make better use of more-traditional treatment modalities.

## IN-HOME PREVENTION AND
## EARLY INTERVENTION PROGRAMS

Sally Provence, a pioneer in the use of home visitation as part of a comprehensive intervention for single, poor, inner-city mothers, was among the first researchers to find that mothers and children who received sustained services from a consistent group of providers through the child's first thirty months of life had positive long-term outcomes in several domains when compared with nonintervention controls. At the end of the Provence intervention, children in the experimental group scored higher in language development; at the time of the five-year follow-up these children demonstrated higher school achievement and better school attendance and were more task oriented. At the five-year follow-up, mothers had fewer additional pregnancies, were more likely to be employed, had improved their socioeconomic status, and made better use of community support resources. After seven and one-half years, mothers had completed more years of education, were more likely to be self-supporting, had more satisfying personal relationships, and had waited longer to have a second child. Mothers who received the intervention were more responsive to the needs of their children and reported a more pleasing relationship with them (Provence, Naylor, and Rescorla, 1983; Seitz, Rosenbaum, and Apfel, 1985).

David Olds, who began his work in Elmira, New York, continues to test his model of nurse-delivered in-home visitation for pregnant and parenting single, poor, primiparous mothers with few social supports in multiple settings throughout the United States. Designed as a preventive public health intervention to affect the quality of parenting, prevent abuse, and improve maternal and infant health, Olds's initial randomized, controlled study in Elmira found that after two years of a structured, curriculum-driven, home visitation program that included parent education, mothers had fewer preterm deliveries, smoked less, and had fewer kidney infections when compared with community controls. Infants had higher birth weights and a 4.86 point increase in I.Q. at 3 and 4 years of age. In addition, the quality of the mother-child relationship was enhanced; mothers provided their children with more play material and used punishment less. The mothers in the Olds study were able to make better use of their own partners and of community supports as well. Children were also seen in the emergency room less frequently and had fewer accidents than the control group. These findings were sustained at the time of follow-up when the children were 15 years old. Reduced incidences of child abuse and neglect were also found at 2 and 15 years. At the time of the 15-year follow-up experimental group children were considerably less likely to have been arrested, use alcohol, smoke cigarettes, or have multiple sexual partners. When the children were 15 years old, mothers in the intervention group were reported as less impaired by drug and alcohol since the birth of the index child (Olds, Robinson, et al., 1999). The initial study was replicated in Memphis, Tennessee, with a primarily urban African American population where many of the effects of the Elmira study were replicated, although the effect size was somewhat smaller. Health-care encounters for injuries and infections were 23 percent lower than in the control group, and the number of hospital days required for serious injuries was significantly less. Olds reports that there were no differences in parents' reports of child behavior problems in either study. An economic analysis conducted by the Rand Corporation found that real economic benefits were accrued by the fourth year of life for low-income children; this finding did not hold for higher socioeconomic status families and married women (Olds and Kitzman, 1993).

Heinicke and Ponce (1999), in a careful review of numerous early intervention studies, found considerable evidence to support the effectiveness of home visitors in improving maternal self-concept and satisfaction and enhancing the responsiveness of the mother to the needs of her infant. The UCLA Family Development Project demonstrated that a randomized home-visiting relationship-based intervention for third-trimester pregnant women who were classified as at high risk for inadequate parenting was able to positively affect experienced partner and family support by infant age 12 months compared to controls (Heinicke et al., 1999). In addition to home visiting, the experimental group participated in a weekly mother-infant group; the controls received regular pediatric follow-up. Children in the intervention group were more securely attached and more autonomous at one year and were encouraged by their mothers to be more task-oriented. The intervention did not affect maternal depression or anxiety, although continued follow-up at year two may produce statistically significant between-group differences. Heinicke points out that the ability to achieve sustained effects with inadequately functioning families depends upon the capacity of the intervention to address the adaptation needs of the parents (ibid.).

The studies reported above demonstrate that sustained, relationship-based, in-home visitation can be effective in improving maternal competence and enhancing maternal capacity to enter into positive relationships, utilize partner and community supports, and attend to issues of self-development. In addition, preventive in-home services support the promotion of the child's autonomy, capacity for exploration, task orientation, and cognition. These studies have also demonstrated the central importance of the sustained relationship between the mother and the service provider in achieving the desired outcomes. The development of a trusting, accepting alliance provides the means through which behavioral changes are able to occur. In this process variables found to be associated with positive outcomes are the duration of the contact between mother and home visitor, the extent of the focus on issues of parenting, the mother's attitude, her willingness to work with the visitor, and her view of the visitor as helpful (Korfmacher, Kitzman, and Olds, 1998).

## FROM CHILD WELFARE PROGRAMS TO TARGETED MENTAL HEALTH TREATMENT: THE ROOTS OF IICAPS

### Family Preservation

Family preservation and support services for families in which children are at high risk of out-of-home placement for reasons of abuse or neglect have existed in the child welfare system for several decades. The Homebuilders program serves as a well-replicated prototype, and variations on the model have proliferated across the United States (Lindblad-Goldberg, Dore, and Stern, 1998). Family preservation programs are time-limited (approximately 12 to 16 weeks), relationship-based, family-focused, child-centered, small-caseload, flexible services that are available to families in the child welfare system 24 hours a day, seven days a week. They are designed to prevent unnecessary out-of-home placements or to promote family reunification by assisting parents to address their own needs and those of their children (Adnopoz and Grigsby, 2002). The majority of referrals to family preservation programs are made by protective service workers who, while concerned about the level of risk to the child existing in the home, believe that with support, the child's parents can provide a safer and more stable environment. Although most studies have shown that placement is prevented for 75 percent to 90 percent of the children receiving services, attempts to determine the effectiveness of family preservation programs have been limited by small effect sizes, the lack of randomized controlled studies, and inadequate program standardization, all of which call into question the adequacy of both the programs and the research methodologies that have been used to evaluate them (Heneghan, Horwitz, and Leventhal, 1996; Burns, Hoagwood, and Mrazek, 1999).

Multiple models of home-based care have been developed to provide targeted interventions for children and families affected by maternal substance abuse, HIV/AIDS, homelessness, and other conditions that place children at risk for instability, loss, and abandonment. The federally funded Abandoned Infants Assistance Program has supported the development of many such comprehensive child welfare programs across the United States (*AIA Best Practices*, 2003). However, child psychiatrists and psychologists are seldom involved in either the development of these programs or the provision of care. Most often the child's parents or caregivers are the primary recipients of the intervention, and services are seldom provided directly to the child.

In the past decade, additional family-focused, in-home services have been tailored specifically to meet the needs of children and adolescents with problems of mental health, delinquency, or substance abuse. Several randomized clinical trials have tested these models and found them to be effective in decreasing problem behaviors, improving family functioning, promoting the recovery of the index child, and reducing the need for more costly out-of-home placements, either in hospitals or in residential programs.

### Multisystemic Therapy (MST)

MST, developed by Henggeler and colleagues (Henggeler et al., 1998), was one of the first in-home programs to identify the youth himself as the primary service recipient, conceptualize the intervention as treatment rather than support, and place the youth and his needs at the center of the treatment plan. MST has informed the development of IICAPS, an intervention that represents an integration of child welfare and medical theories and practices.

A manualized, intensive, home-based therapeutic-approach, multisystemic therapy developed by Henggeler and his associates, MST has demonstrated its effectiveness with chronic juvenile offenders, adolescent sex offenders, and substance-abusing delinquents. MST directly addresses the interpersonal and systemic factors that are associated with adolescent antisocial behavior (Henggeler and Borduin, 1990) and considers the child's view of his world as well as the direct and persistent influence of his family, peer, and school environments. Sessions are held frequently in the child's home and in the community; services are time-limited and are designed to empower parents to understand and manage behavioral crises as they may arise following the intervention. The Missouri Delinquency Project examined the long-term effects of MST on the prevention of criminal activity in a sample of predominantly serious juvenile offenders by comparing MST with individual therapy, and demonstrated positive effects on perceived family relations, family interactions, parental symptomology, interfamilial conflict, and youths' behavioral problems. The intervention also produced long-term changes in youths' criminal behaviors. Central to the success of MST has been an understanding of the familial and social contexts in which youths function and by which they are strongly influenced, coupled with a willingness to address the contextual issues within a structured curriculum. Borduin suggests that improved family functioning, a result of in-home and community services, was the primary influence on the reduction of criminal behavior in the Missouri study (Borduin et al., 1995).

Henggeler and his colleagues (Henggeler et al., 1999) have reported on a study to determine whether MST could be modified effectively for use with youths presenting with psychiatric emergencies and utilized as an alternative to psychiatric hospitalization. Based on the hypotheses that the child's family plays a central role in predicting and preventing the need for hospitalization, and that behaviors are socially and ecologically influenced, Henggeler designed and tested an intervention for children ages 10–17 who were approved for emergency psychiatric hospitalization at the Medical University of South Carolina. These youths were randomly assigned to either an MST experimental condition or to hospitalization and aftercare. Services were provided in the homes of immediate family, relatives, or friends and in community shelters, respite beds, or hospitals. Caseloads were reduced from the MST standard of five families per clinician to three. Children in the experimental group had judicious and controlled access to community resources, including hospitalization and therapeutic foster care. Children in the control group received treatment as usual, often utilizing some of the same resources (Henggeler et al., 1999).

Henggeler et al. (ibid.) reported that MST was at least as effective as, and in some cases more effective than, emergency psychiatric hospitalization at decreasing child symptomology. Rates of decreased internalizing problems were similar across the two conditions; MST was more effective in decreasing rates of externalizing symptoms. Youths in the control condition reported increased self-esteem; families in the experimental condition showed improved cohesion and increased structure. Henggeler et al. noted that the treatment of youths with serious psychiatric problems and their families presents greater complexity and problem severity than was expected on the basis of their previous work. Further study, some of which is already in progress, is needed to address the issues raised by this evaluation (ibid.).

**Wraparound**

The wraparound concept of services that place the child in the context of his family and his broader social ecology emerged from the Child and Adolescent Service System Program (CASSP). CASSP was dedicated to the creation of interagency collaborations; community-based, advocacy-oriented systems of care; and the expansion of parental decision making and involvement to meet the multisystemic needs of children with serious emotional disturbances (Woolston et al., 1998). Theoretically based in human ecology, wraparound stresses unconditional care and assumes that changes in the environment will foster changes that persist over time for children, families, and communities. Wraparound is a strength-based process of intervention that values parental empowerment, culturally competent providers, group process, and the use of natural supports to augment professional involvement. Outcomes are measured against goals established by the family. Wraparound teams are led by a bachelor's-level resource coordinator who does not provide clinical care. As a result the quality of clinical care is dependent upon the quality of the resources available in the local system of care. Wraparound services have no time limit, are available 24 hours a day, seven days a week, and are provided in home, school, clinic, and community. In comparing the effects of MST and wraparound, Burns and fellow researchers found a need for randomized effectiveness trials to demonstrate the effectiveness of wraparound in light of the speed of its national replication, the observable variations in its implementation, its potential for cost savings, and the increasing availability of standards and measures of fidelity (Burns et al., 2000).

**THE EMERGENCE OF IICAPS**

IICAPS reflects the further refinement of in-home services for the treatment of children with serious psychiatric disturbances. It is firmly rooted in the history of legislatively supported, theoretically grounded services for children whose illness places them at risk for costly treatments necessitating lengthy separation from their families and communities. IICAPS has been welcomed by families because of its insistence on family leadership and involvement and its interest in the protection of family cohesion. It has been embraced by the Connecticut Department of Children and Families and endorsed by managed-care companies as a psychiatric service that is effective both clinically and fiscally. It provides a model of clinical care for children and families in the real world that enables them to experience success in meeting the potentially achievable treatment goals they set for themselves and their children. The expectations regarding outcomes are modest and shaped by realistic assessment of the child's and family's potential. The desired child and family behaviors are those that will maintain the child safely in his home and community and reduce the need for hospitalization. For these reasons IICAPS shows strong promise as a treatment model that has already demonstrated its ability to address the crises facing the mental health system today. The 14 Connecticut IICAPS treatment sites show preliminary evidence of reducing dependence on resources such as psychiatric hospitals, while improving child functioning. Although a randomized study of its effectiveness has not been completed, there is much to recommend it as a treatment of choice.

In addition to offering a specific model of treatment for children with SED and their families, the structured format that defines an IICAPS intervention can be applied more widely in the service of family-focused, skill-centered care. This volume describes and illustrates the concepts, assumptions, and specific tools that characterize the IICAPS treatment model and can inform the planning and delivery of behavioral health services regardless of the model through which services are delivered.

# Chapter 2 Introduction to IICAPS

The Intensive In-Home Child and Adolescent Psychiatric Service (Woolston et al., 1998) is a home-based psychiatric treatment whose overarching goal is to improve the developmental trajectory of children and adolescents with SED while reducing or preventing the need for institution-based treatments. The children and families served by IICAPS are either at risk for requiring institution-based care, unable to be discharged from such care without intensive treatment and support, or sufficiently unresponsive to outpatient services that their basic developmental achievements are compromised.

To accomplish its mission IICAPS utilizes a multidimensional, multisystemic approach that considers the child's specific psychiatric disorder, the parenting practices and patterns of family functioning, and the broader ecological context of the child's life. IICAPS interventions address the primary domains of the child's life and establish goals in each of them. The IICAPS model is informed by concepts and findings from developmental psychopathology that, when applied as part of the intervention, further the understanding of the multiple determinants that keep children and family members stuck at their current level of dysfunction.

A two-person clinical team composed of a license-eligible or licensed mental health provider and a bachelor's-level mental health clinician provide all IICAPS services. This team provides a continuum of psychiatric and other comprehensive services to the child and family in their home and community. In addition to regular weekly meetings with a supervisor, a senior mental health clinician, each IICAPS team is expected to present assessment and ongoing treatment information every three weeks in multidisciplinary staff rounds that are co-led by a child and adolescent psychiatrist who serves as medical director of the IICAPS intervention.

Fidelity to the IICAPS model is measured by the degree of adherence demonstrated by the team and supervisor to the fundamental structures that differentiate IICAPS from other in-home service models. These structures, IICAPS Principles, Concepts, and Tools, provide a nested set of constructs that move from the general (Principles) to the specific (Tools) and serve to mark progress, identify barriers to treatment, and promote active engagement and partnership with families throughout the life of the intervention. Each element of these fundamental structures is designed to provide a flexible framework to simultaneously guide the IICAPS intervention and permit quantitative measurement of adherence to the IICAPS model.

### PROGRAM HISTORY

IICAPS was developed by the authors, members of the faculty of the Yale Child Study Center, in 1996 in response to the challenges and opportunities created in Connecticut by the shift in Medicaid-funded services from a fee-for-service payment model to managed care. The shift to managed Medicaid precipitated a rapid drop in lengths of stay on psychiatric in-patient services and a concomitant rise in both psychiatric in-patient readmissions and emergency department psychiatric consultations. However, the shift away from fee-for-service funding also presented opportunities for managed-care companies to become more flexible in their approach to the funding of service provision and more open to the purchase of services that showed promise of caring for children with SED more creatively and with greater cost effectiveness.

In this environment IICAPS was conceptualized as an intervention that was able to combine the benefits of intensive, psychiatric in-patient treatment with the holistic, ecological, family-centered, child-welfare-oriented approach of clinically informed in-home family preservation. Drawing upon their expertise in each of these approaches, and with the support of both the Yale School of Medicine and a managed-care company that agreed to pay negotiated charges for children whose needs met medical necessity criteria, Yale Child Study Center faculty members created the first IICAPS team in 1996.

From 1996 to 2001, IICAPS consisted of a single program at the Child Study Center, initially staffed by teams paid on a fee-for-service basis and trained and supervised by the authors and their colleagues. In 2002, Connecticut's Department of Children and Families (DCF), the integrated Connecticut state agency responsible for child protective, juvenile justice and child mental health services, contracted with the IICAPS developers to implement IICAPS in 16 additional sites throughout Connecticut. IICAPS was seen as one of the cornerstones of KidCare, an innovative, publicly supported, statewide mental health initiative for children with SED that was designed to maintain and treat children and families in their homes and communities whenever possible (Connecticut Department of Children and Families, 2003).

The statewide implementation of IICAPS was both a challenge and the impetus for development of an IICAPS treatment manual and associated training, supervision, consultation, and network development protocols. By 2004 more than 500 children and families had received or were receiving IICAPS treatment in Connecticut. The initial quality-assurance data indicated that institution-based service utilization was substantially reduced as compared to a similar sample of children with SED from a nearby state where IICAPS was not available (Blader, 2004).

## THEORETICAL ASSUMPTIONS

All aspects of the IICAPS intervention are grounded in three broad sets of constructs: developmental psychopathology; psychology of motivation, action, and problem solving; and systems of care philosophy. Concepts from developmental psychopathology further the understanding of the child who is the focus of the IICAPS treatment. The youths whom IICAPS treats are psychiatrically disturbed and often live in ongoing psychosocial adversity that compounds psychopathology, inhibits effective treatment, and/or is a contributing cause of the psychiatric disturbance. The psychology of motivation, action, and problem solving guides the treatment process with the family members involved by enhancing ongoing engagement and effective problem solving. The iterative process that is central to the IICAPS model is reflected in the creation and implementation of a treatment plan that is specific to the strengths and vulnerabilities of each child and family member. Development of the treatment plan begins with the identification by the family members of the behavior that puts the identified child at risk for requiring institution-based treatment. Subsequently the family members and treatment team enumerate the salient vulnerabilities and strengths that maintain the problematic behavior. The IICAPS model then guides the family through the process of building upon its strengths and reducing recognized vulnerabilities to attain the goals that the family members set for themselves. Each component of this treatment process is constructed so as to maximize engagement. This ongoing engagement process is exemplified by capturing each identified problem, goal, and step of treatment in the language of the family members. System of care philosophy directs the multisystemic approach to IICAPS. This philosophy is consistent with constructs from developmental psychopathology that underscore the crucial nature of the child's entire social ecology in creating and ameliorating serious emotional disturbance.

### Developmental Psychopathology, Transactional Risk Model, and Gene-Environment Interaction Paradigm for Development

Developmental psychopathology is an overarching theory of developmental processes and derailments that incorporates and, in turn, helps explicate and merge many more-specific developmental models. It differs from many of these models in that it is continually empirically validated and describes complex causal relationships among various factors that result in psychopathological outcomes. The theory dictates that treatment interventions for children with severe psychiatric impairments should also operate in multiple interacting domains. As a result, developmental psychopathology guides treaters to match specific interventions to the particular needs of each child and family.

Studies of developmental psychopathology have shown that the developmental trajectory of each individual is a complex phenomenon that is best described by the transactional risk model of development (Sameroff and Fiese, 1989; Woolston, 1989; Cicchetti, Rogosch, and Toth, 1997; Cicchetti and Toth, 1999). In essence, the transactional risk model posits that development occurs through complex interactions between and among genetic and epigenetic substrates and their products, individual behavior and psychology, and environmental stimuli that are the constituents of optimal development as well as vulnerable elements that are risks for deficient developmental outcomes. Any one of these elements may contribute to psychopathology or resilience in an interactive fashion.

The transactional risk model is composed of several constructs. First, it proposes that developmental trajectories, or outcomes measured at any particular point in time, are probabilistic rather than deterministic. This construct of *probabilistic outcomes* is in direct opposition to several historically important and diverse models of development such as psychoanalytic theory, behaviorism, and family systems theory. As different as each of these theories is, each posits that the initial characteristics of an individual's development will be highly predictive of later outcomes. In contrast, the transactional risk model proposes that developmental outcomes are the result of extremely complex interactions from which many different developmental outcomes can be expected. A single, common outcome can result from multiple initial conditions (equifinality), while a range of different outcomes can result from apparently identical initial conditions (multifinality).

The second construct of the transactional risk model posits that the probabilistic nature of developmental outcomes results from the complex set of interactions that occur among each individual's strengths and vulnerabilities with varying effects. Such complex interactions are described by the concept of *risk and protective factor accrual.* In this context the effect of the interaction between each child's strengths and vulnerabilities may be additive and may have immediate, delayed, or latent influence. Many studies have shown that the simultaneous presence of multiple risk factors can exert a much more deleterious influence on development than a single risk factor. Similarly the presence of multiple protective factors may neutralize the negative influence of one or more risk factors (Garmezy, 1983). The phenomenon of accrual of influence may well have multiple origins. Some factors may alter the organism so that it becomes more vulnerable to the influence of other factors that by themselves would be unlikely to produce a negative effect. For example, the children served by IICAPS may suffer from the additive effects of living in families affected by low-income status, chronic parental mental and/or physical illness, unemployment, and instability. However, while there are sets of risk and protective factors that may increase the odds of certain outcomes, these outcomes are never certain.

The third construct of the transactional risk model posits that neither the individual nor the environment is a passive element in the course of development but rather continuously engages in active, *bidirectional interaction.* The individual's personal environment, or microsystem, includes elements such as the child's inner world, family, friends, physical environment, neighborhood, and school, which continually interact. Consistent with the construct of bidirectionality, the interaction of these elements forms the core of each child's life experience. The microsystem thus formed for each child is conceptualized as a nested set of interrelated systems ranging from the biological to the social, whose interactions are described by general systems theory (Von Bertalanffy, 1968).

The apparently probabilistic nature of development described by the transactional risk model interacts with ontogenesis, the regular, patterned, unfolding of development. Ontogenesis describes the phases in which each child experiences new developmental opportunities that stimulate new adaptations (Cicchetti, Rogosch, and Toth, 1997). The degree and quality of adaptation to these stage- and phase-salient tasks influence how a particular developmental issue is incorporated into the child's psychological, neurological, and physical organization. Positive adaptation contributes to *competence,* whereas compromised resolution increases the likelihood of *incompetence.* However, the outcome is always determined in a probabilistic, not deterministic, fashion.

Despite the probabilistic nature of developmental outcomes, some stages offer absolute or relatively unique opportunities for developmental organization. Stages that appear to offer absolutely unique developmental opportunities are called critical periods, while those that offer almost unique opportunities are called sensitive periods. For example, a significant body of experimental data supports the premise that in mammals, the neonatal period is a critical period for the organization of the visual cortex. If a mammal is deprived of meaningful visual stimuli during this period, or, more specifically, if the visual cortex is deprived of such stimuli, the visual cortex is rendered permanently unable to process visual information. In contrast, sensitive periods are less well defined but remain a crucial time for specific developmental organization. For example, in social primates, the developmental periods of infancy and toddlerhood are important times for the acquisition of species-specific socialization skills and attachment mechanisms. As shown by Harlow and Harlow (1962), social primates that have been deprived of positive, species-specific social experiences during this sensitive period had an array of social skill deficits for the remainder of their lives. However, the degree and severity of these deficits can vary depending upon the exact time and nature of the inadequate social experience as well as the individual's life experiences after the sensitive period is past.

The concepts and presumptions that inform the developmental theories of ontogenesis, risk accrual, probabilistic developmental outcomes, and bidirectionality of development have now been enriched and extended by the gene-environment interaction (G × E) paradigm for development (Moffitt, 2005). The G × E paradigm for development posits that relatively minor and common variations in genes interact in complex ways with developmental experiences to influence, but not guarantee, the development of stable constellations of functioning, so-called behavioral phenotypes. Currently the best-studied behavioral phenotype is antisocial behavior (Moffitt, 2005). Caspi and colleagues (2002) have reported a study that used a large community sample followed longitudinally from birth to young adulthood. The study included careful monitoring of the psychosocial environment and behaviors of the subjects as well as evaluating variations of specific genes. Specifically the researchers looked at the relationship between the effects of child maltreatment and variations of a gene (alleles) that encoded for the neurotransmitter-metabolizing enzyme monoamine oxidase A (MAOA). One allele of MAOA gene produced a relatively low-activity enzyme while the other produced MAOA with higher activity. Since the gene for MAOA is on the X chromosome, boys have one copy while girls have two, one of which is randomly inactivated throughout the body. Since girls therefore have a much more complex expression of MAOA gene, they were not studied in this report. Only the boys with the combination of both the low-activity MAOA allele and the experience of maltreatment displayed antisocial behaviors by age 26 years. Boys with the low-activity MAOA but no exposure to maltreatment had the same, low rate of antisocial behaviors by age 26 years as boys who had high-activity MAOA and maltreatment or no maltreatment experience. Thus, neither the presence of the low-activity MAOA allele nor the experience of maltreatment in childhood by itself increased the risk of antisocial behavior, but the combination of the two factors did cause a significant increase in antisocial behavior. In contrast, the presence of the high-activity MAOA allele appeared to protect against the tendency for childhood maltreatment to be associated with antisocial behavior as a young adult. Importantly, these findings have been replicated and extended by an independent research team studying a different sample (Foley et al., 2004).

These studies illustrate the potential the G × E interaction paradigm has for illuminating the complexities of the developmental process, including the probabilistic and interactive nature of development. Moffitt (2005) emphasizes that a particular gene, or gene allele, is related not to a disorder but rather to the response of individual organisms to environmental risk. The environmental risk is not a static phenomenon but rather a cascade (Caspi and Moffitt, 1995) that, after being initiated, can have "consequences of its own, cutting off opportunities to develop healthy behaviors, promoting the persistence of pathological behavior, and exacerbating its seriousness" (Moffitt, 2005, p. 547). Interrupting this "cascade" resonating through the child's psychosocial world then becomes the focus of interventions to limit the severity and persistence of behavioral phenotypes or disorders.

While study of the G × E paradigm is just beginning, data derived from the heuristic constructs of the transactional risk model and ontogenesis can guide interventions for serious emotional disturbance in children. For example, it is known that there are varying times throughout the course of development when children's vulnerability to environmental risk factors and adverse experiences may be heightened. Phase-specific issues, brain development, and other factors affect children differentially depending on their age and stage of development. For example, infants and toddlers are especially vulnerable to long separations from primary caretakers; school-age children are particularly sensitive to issues of intellectual and physical prowess, and adolescents to issues related to body image, peer acceptance, and sexuality.

Development, with its sensitive periods, does not end with adolescence but continues throughout the life cycle. IICAPS interventions incorporate these developmental constructs into each child's treatment plan not only by addressing the identified child's developmental needs but also by considering the needs of all other members of his family. In addition, by intervening in the four specific domains that are germane to each child's life and in which the child may have difficulties, IICAPS treatment focuses upon improving the fit between the child's needs and his/her ecology. By understanding the contributions of various factors to the unfolding of the child's development, interventions can be directed toward modification of those specific elements that inhibit optimum developmental progress.

### Family Members Lead the Way:
### Engagement and Problem-Solving Therapy

Only the child and important family members have the knowledge and power to change the crucial components of the cascade of environmental risk factors so that the trajectory of the child's SED can be improved. This is a core construct of the IICAPS intervention. Authentic engagement of family members in the treatment process is considered the sine qua non for any effective intervention. In the past decade there have been significant advances in the understanding and improvement of engagement in behavioral health services (McKay and Bannon, 2004). Engagement in child mental health services has been divided into two specific steps: initial attendance and ongoing engagement (McKay et al., 1998). In the child mental health literature, treatment of antisocial behavior has provided the most useful information related to the understanding of ongoing engagement. For example, enhanced family treatment (Prinz and Miller, 1994) and multisystemic therapy (Henggeler et al., 1996) have described an explicit ecological approach to identify and address barriers to ongoing participation in treatment. An extension of this problem-solving approach has been used in parent management training to address other life stressors with which parents struggle (Kazdin and Whitley, 2003).

In IICAPS intervention, engagement in the treatment process is an ongoing strategy that is supported by and included in the IICAPS treatment structures. This active, ongoing engagement occurs via structures and mechanisms designed not only to remove barriers to entrance into treatment but also to enhance treatment effectiveness. The IICAPS structures are consistent with the concepts articulated in the psychology of motivation and action (Oettingen and Gollwitzer, 2001) in relation to goal setting (Oettingen, 2000), goal implementation (Gollwitzer, 1999), and mental contrasting (Oettingen, 1999). These concepts are embedded in each step that moves from engagement to treatment planning, from treatment planning to treatment implementation, and from treatment implementation to treatment review. In addition, the treatment process itself is guided by problem-solving training. Problem-solving training has a large literature in its own right that has demonstrated its effectiveness as an accepted approach to a multitude of issues (D'Zurilla and Nezu, 1999). Principles from problem-solving training are ideally suited to supporting ongoing engagement between the family and the therapist because they place considerable emphasis on enhancing social competence. Not only does this approach require authentic participation between the therapist and client, but it is inherently empowering as well.

While IICAPS places emphasis on the initial phase of engagement, the IICAPS structures are intended to promote and support engagement throughout the course of the intervention. These IICAPS structures are characterized by a series of tasks performed mutually by the IICAPS team and family members that lead to creation of a treatment plan, the effective implementation of the treatment plan, and, finally, the development of a coauthored treatment summary and discharge plan. Each step of this process is informed by the concepts of problem-solving training.

### Systems of Care

While IICAPS is informed by theories of developmental psychology and psychopathology at the level of individual children and families, it is also influenced by principles and concepts pertaining to the theory of system of care that operate on a broader social level. The system of care concept was developed by a consensus of mental health professionals, advocates, and policy makers (Osher et al., 1999; Weisz, Huey, and Weersing, 1998). The widely accepted principles that inform the concept of systems of care have had a significant influence on current professional practice, services, training, and public mental health policy for children with SED throughout the United States and beyond. Key constructs of systems of care place a high value on specific service characteristics. Among the most prized of these are (1) that interventions are family driven and reflective of the child and family's wishes as well as their needs, and (2) that interventions address the primary areas of the child's life in a manner that is culturally and linguistically responsive. In addition, interventions within the system of care models are expected to be sensitive to individual and family differences and informed by the family's identification of the strengths upon which they can draw to address the vulnerabilities that perpetuate the child's problems. Systems of care principles staunchly maintain that families must be full partners in the work of treatment. Being full partners requires family members to become actively engaged as members of the treatment team; conversely, enlisting the family as full partners requires that the family be treated with respect, cooperation, and collaboration.

### APPLICATION TO IICAPS

Consistent with constructs from the transactional risk model, ontogenesis, problem-solving training, and systems of care theory, the IICAPS intervention begins with an assessment of the interacting strengths and vulnerabilities in the child's microsystem that are either inhibiting or promoting his/her healthy development. After the initial assessment, the IICAPS model requires the development of a treatment plan with the child and family members as equal partners in the process that will lead to increased strengths and decreased vulnerabilities in the child's microsystem. Involving the child and family members as equal partners in all Phases of IICAPS is essential to the intervention for the following reasons. First, given the complexity of development, only the child and family members have intimate knowledge of those aspects of the child's functioning that must be changed for the child's developmental trajectory to be improved. They are the most qualified to identify the mechanisms that might best be employed to bring about the changes they desire. Second, only the child and important family members have the power to create meaningful changes in their microsystem. Third, only the child and family members have the capacity to internalize the elements that are expected to lead to an improved trajectory so that they can continue to influence the child's functioning after the IICAPS intervention has concluded

### OVERARCHING IICAPS GOAL AND PARAMETERS

The children with SED appropriate for referral for IICAPS intervention present with complicated and chronic problems that threaten to derail their healthy development and disturb family functioning. The overarching goal of an IICAPS intervention is to reduce the child's risk of requiring institution-based treatment by optimizing the fit between the child and his microsystem. When an IICAPS team and family members work together to create new, stable, health-promoting interactions in the child's microsystem, the child is more likely to move toward recovery. The IICAPS goal is accomplished when this level of stabilization occurs and the child is no longer reliant on the external structure of the institution or hospital for safety or containment. Almost all children and families served by IICAPS will require a variety of ongoing psychiatric, educational, and social services after the IICAPS intervention is finished. In fact one essential element of IICAPS action is to improve the fit between the family members and the other elements of the microsystem so that the family members can reliably and effectively access needed community- and clinic-based services.

The desire to curtail utilization of hospital and institutional placements while increasing the access to and availability of community-based services is based upon the recognized limitations of restrictive care. Among these limitations is the fact that institutionally based treatments are extremely expensive. Since funding for children's mental health services is generally a zero-sum allocation, every dollar spent on one category of care generally means that additional dollars are not available for other funding categories. When increased amounts of funding are devoted to removing children from their homes and communities and placing them in restrictive, institution-based care, fewer funds are available for less-restrictive, community-based care. As a result, community-based care may be less available. In such communities, children may be kept in institution-based care longer than needed to achieve greater symptom improvement.

When and if symptom improvement is achieved children may be discharged to a community setting that will have few services to support the maintenance of their gains. This process can be, and frequently is, self-perpetuating, so that more and more youths spend longer and longer time in institutions.

A second limitation to hospital- and other institution-based care is that it places the child in an abnormal psychosocial world that heightens his risk of further disrupted development. Institutionalization is the phenomenon of compromised individual development as a sequela of living in a restrictive environment. Although institutionalization occurs in adults after they have lived in restrictive placements for long periods, it occurs much more rapidly for youths, for whom time is an important element in the developmental process.

A third limitation of institution-based care is the lack of empirical support for either its efficacy or safety. Performing a randomized controlled study of the effectiveness of institution-based care is extremely challenging. Finding an ethical alternative to serve as a randomized control arm of a study presents a considerable problem for investigators, since the youths involved are likely to be experiencing severe, even life-threatening psychiatric symptomology. Thus, while there are substantive reasons for the lack of such empirical support for the efficacy and safety of institution-based care, the absence of such data requires even greater caution about endorsing this treatment option. Removal from family and community should become the treatment of choice only when less-restrictive alternatives are too dangerous and the probability that the child cannot remain safely in his home and community appears to be too great.

A fourth limitation of hospital and other institution-based care relates to the lack of preparation provided for families prior to their child's return to home and community. Most frequently institution-based treatments focus on altering the child's psychiatric symptoms by treatments emanating from elements within the institution. Having significant interaction with family members is difficult to accomplish and may seem contrary to the purpose of removing the youth from the environment in which the problems developed. Even when family members are frequently engaged with the youth in the institution, the nature of the involvement is distorted by the fact that it occurs within the institutional setting rather than in the real-world environment of the home and community.

Within its stated overarching goal, IICAPS embraces two treatment parameters. First, IICAPS is based upon empowering family members to optimize the fit between the child and her microsystem. At each step of the intervention the family members are the leading edge of the treatment process. IICAPS is fully voluntary; all work reflects the language, perceptions, and understanding of the family members; family members must understand, coauthor, and regularly evaluate each component of the intervention. Second, IICAPS is a time-limited intervention with clearly defined Phases of treatment. The time-limited nature of the intervention helps keep both the IICAPS team and family members realistic about the goals of treatment. IICAPS treatment is focused on specific goals that can be accomplished by the family members. While IICAPS treatment can occur only as a result of the work of the family members, they are not expected to do this work by themselves. For the vast majority of children and families, the successful end of treatment is marked by the child's and family's having stable connections with a variety of professional services and naturalistic supports and that together create an environment able to sustain the child in his home setting. These services and supports frequently include outpatient pharmacotherapy and psychotherapy, new and individualized school plans, and involvement in supportive after-school activities.

## CHILDREN AND FAMILIES SERVED BY IICAPS

Children and adolescents who are expected to benefit from IICAPS have two simultaneous and interacting sets of vulnerabilities or impairment criteria functionally related to themselves and their families. First, these youths suffer with significant psychiatric disorders. The types of psychiatric disorders frequently found in the IICAPS treatment population range from severe, childhood-onset, neuropsychiatric disorders, such as Schizophrenia, major mood disorders, or pervasive developmental disorders to disorders that are the sequelae of early trauma and disruptions of attachment. These latter disorders may present as severe dysregulations of mood, anxiety, aggression, and impulse control as well as more classic post-traumatic stress disorders.

Most children who receive IICAPS services have a combination of neuropsychiatrically based and stress- and/or trauma-induced disorders. A growing literature from developmental psychopathology and from behavioral health treatment provides numerous, specific, and empirically demonstrated effective interventions for various serious behavioral health disorders of children and youths (Weersing and Weisz, 2002). Among these interventions are psychopharmacotherapy for symptoms of attention-deficit/hyperactivity disorders, mood disorders, psychotic disorders, and the like; cognitive-behavioral therapy (CBT) for anxiety, depression, and post-traumatic stress disorder; parent management training (PMT) for disruptive behavior disorders; and supportive psychotherapy for adjustment disorders.

Pharmacologic and psychosocial interventions have been shown to have a significant effect on improvements in functioning and reduction of child symptomology. All IICAPS teams are expected to be familiar with these therapies and sufficiently competent to initiate them or to facilitate their initiation when appropriate to the child's psychopathology either directly or in conjunction with other outpatient treaters. Even so, these interventions will not be successful if they are provided in isolation from the reality of the child's world. To achieve positive treatment effects the child must reside in a minimally adequate psychosocial environment with caregivers able to respond to his needs.

Among the children and youths who may be referred appropriately for IICAPS interventions are those whose families have been unable to provide the level of care and understanding that they require to be maintained safely at home. The factors that inhibit the capacity of parents to meet the physical and psychological needs of their children constitute the second set of vulnerabilities that interact with and possibly exacerbate the effect of the child's own individual disorder. Rutter (Quinton and Rutter, 1984) and others have identified some of the many factors that may compromise the ability of families to provide a safe, psychosocial home environment. Key among them are parental neuropsychiatric disorders, as well as parental difficulties such as limited cognition, severe, chronic stress-induced disorders, chronic physical illness, and addiction to drugs and/or alcohol. The psychosocial conditions associated with poverty, such as inadequate housing, lack of employment, social isolation, and marginalization, and limited access to treatment further limit the family's ability to provide appropriate care.

This dilemma posed by a child's behavioral health treatment's being thwarted by an inadequate psychosocial environment is one of the rationales used to justify the placement of children in institution-based treatments. Indeed, there are times when the nature of a child's disorder, coupled with the intractable deficits in the capacity of the child's microsystem, favors the selection of institutional treatment. More frequently, institutional treatment is chosen because there appear to be no other viable alternatives.

In Connecticut IICAPS has been accepted as an alternative to institution-based treatment with the capacity to alter the fit between the child and his environment by improving the family's ability to recognize and meet his needs. Interventions take place across the four Domains that are central to the IICAPS ecologic approach; the child, the family, the school, and the other systems with which the child and family regularly interact. Goals across these Domains may include a decrease in the child's psychiatric symptoms, the remediation of problematic parenting practices, improvement in the child's educational programming, and a reduction of the environmental factors that contribute to the child's psychosocial adversity.

In addition to meeting inclusionary criteria of serious psychiatric illness and inadequate family environment, children and adolescents eligible for IICAPS treatment must meet three other criteria. First, IICAPS interventions cannot be implemented without the voluntary agreement of the child's parent or legal guardian to be a full participant in the work of treatment, a position consistent with the theories that inform IICAPS intervention. Second, there must be an identified funding entity, generally a managed-care company that recognizes the extent of the child's or adolescent's illness and is willing to join with the IICAPS team through the mechanism of reimbursement. Ideally the funding entity has responsibility and authority for paying for any and all behavioral health treatments for the youth. This responsibility and authority enhance the funder's motivation and ability to facilitate the creation of a stable set of services that may begin with the initiation of IICAPS and continue after the IICAPS treatment is finished.

The third inclusionary criterion is that the youth and family live in a home environment that is sufficiently accessible to the IICAPS staff to permit intensive, home-based work. The requirement that the child's family environment be open and available to the IICAPS team is consistent with the aim to understand the child and family's microsystem well enough that meaningful changes can be initiated. If a family is living in an environment over which they have little or no control (such as a homeless shelter or "on the street"), it will not be feasible to bring about meaningful changes in the child's microsystem. If a family lives in a home that is not available for frequent home visits and crisis emergency intervention, then IICAPS treatment cannot be implemented.

## IICAPS: MULTIPLE ORGANIZATIONAL LEVELS

IICAPS interventions consist of multiple nested and interdependent functional levels of organization. The child and his/her environment or microsystem constitute the case level, the central level of organization for the intervention.

Much of the work of IICAPS occurs at this level, in which services, such as psychiatric assessment and treatment, intensive care management, and crisis intervention are provided. These types of services are fully integrated into the IICAPS model and are consistent with the program's overarching goals. The psychiatric assessment of the identified child and other family members, when indicated, is expected to lead to improved understanding of the child's psychiatric disorder and amelioration of the dangerous behaviors in which he may be engaged. Simultaneously the assessment may also reveal the limitations and incapacities of the parents. The provision of intensive care management may bring about changes within the family that are small but sufficiently important to enable them to enter into the work of making larger, more lasting changes in their microsystem.

Because staff is available to the child and family 24 hours per day, seven days per week, to handle crises as they appear, the likelihood that a sudden but transient episode of problematic behavior will result in institution-based care is reduced significantly. Utilization of these three types of interventions (psychiatric assessment and treatment of the child, intensive care management, and crisis intervention) guides the child, the family, and the IICAPS team through the critical processes of problem identification, treatment plan development, plan implementation, and continual plan refinement. This organizational structure at the case level is designed to promote the attainment of the treatment goals and the achievement of the ultimate aim of maintaining the child safely in his home.

The second level of IICAPS organization focuses upon the quality of the relationship that exists between the master's-prepared and the bachelor's-prepared IICAPS team members who together provide the clinical care for IICAPS children and their families. The team model was selected as the design of choice by the IICAPS model developers largely because the clinical and emotional demands associated with intensive home-based intervention are likely to overwhelm a single practitioner. As the primary agents of IICAPS services, team members carry the burden of implementing the treatment model in adherence to the training manual. In recognition of these responsibilities and in acknowledgment that many practitioners are working in the field of home-based services for the first time, IICAPS requires consistent, frequent supervision. IICAPS administrators and supervisors must share a commitment to creating multiple opportunities for ongoing training and skill development. Chapter 7 contains a more detailed description of IICAPS staff organization.

# Chapter 3 Working with
# Families in Their Own Homes

## A FAMILY-FOCUSED APPROACH

Behavioral health interventions offered to children and families in their own homes incorporate many of the theories, principles, and constructs that inform all clinically competent care for children with SED regardless of the setting in which they are applied. However, working with children and families in the home requires knowledge, theoretical orientation, and skills that differentiate home-based treatment from treatment in a traditional outpatient setting. In this chapter we discuss the importance of family participation in the treatment of children with SED and the unique opportunities presented when the treatment site is, in fact, the family living room or kitchen and when the family therapy session includes extended family members and others who play significant roles in the family.

The family has long been recognized as the most effective long-term institution for raising children (Goldstein et al., 1996). Solnit (1976) has described the family as "the bridge from the past to the future." The family provides its members with a sense of being rooted in time, place, history, and culture. The family's functional capacity exerts a central influence on each child's ability to adapt to and cope with the vicissitudes of life. Parental capacity to think reflectively, to understand the child as a separate individual with his own strengths, needs, vulnerabilities, wishes, and feelings, is associated with the child's sense of competency (Tebes, Kaufman, Adnopoz, and Racusin, 1999). Theoretical constructs derived from social ecology and developmental psychopathology support the view that each child's functioning is the result of the continuous interactions between his/her innate structural capacities and the systems that make up his social environment (Woolston et al., 1998).

The central role of the family in human development has been supported both by clinical experience and by research in developmental psychopathology. Adequately functioning families provide the experiences that are essential to support the human developmental processes: nurturance, safety, stability, and a sense of being wanted. Consistent nurturing and responsive relationships between children and their family caregivers enable children to feel secure in their environment and promote their capacity for growth and maturation throughout all developmental stages and phases. Families not only serve as nurturers and satisfiers of need; they also are the primary means through which the child receives information about his or her world. Families are responsible for establishing the limits and boundaries that promote each child's sense of security and safety. Adequately functioning families can promote exploration and creativity and lend support to the child's physical, social, and academic progress. Through both spoken and unspoken communication, families influence the child's view of himself, his expectations of himself, and the ways in which he responds to the world in which he lives. Because families are the primary source of information about their own history, culture, and belief system, they provide children with a sense of the past. At the same time, the family's existence over time projects hope for the child's future.

Consonant with the transactional risk model described earlier in this volume, the interaction among family members is complex and dynamic. Each family member continually acts and is acted upon by all other members. In this way, families exert significant influence on the growth and development of their members and promote or inhibit the ability of children to adapt and cope with both expectable and unforeseen challenges. Disruption of parent-child relationships can interfere with normative developmental processes and profoundly influence the child's sense of self-adequacy and his capacity for intimacy. Following the precepts of developmental psychopathology, just as healthy development is promoted by positive family interactions, so, too, the recovery of children with SED is improved when family members are involved in the process. When important family members are actively involved, the problems occurring within the family that are affecting the child's illness may be addressed openly.

Despite being committed to the child's recovery, many families may experience significant barriers to using community-based treatments. Some families are not sufficiently organized to access traditional outpatient services. Others are coping with multiple stressors and personal demands that adversely affect their ability to adhere to appointment schedules and prescribed treatment protocols. Family members may find the physical setting of clinic-based treatment problematic but may be willing to become engaged in family-oriented treatments provided in the more familiar environment of their home.

In these and similar situations, home-based treatment offers children, youths, and families several advantages over clinic-based care. For some family members the home visit is less stressful than coming to an outpatient setting. For others, bringing services into the home facilitates the inclusion of all members of the family system in the treatment and promotes their contribution to the process of returning the child to healthier functioning. With the venue of service moved from the clinician's office to the home, the balance of power is shifted from the clinician to the family. By the act of entering the child's home and neighborhood, the clinical providers signal acceptance of the family's lifestyle and beliefs. Scheduling meetings at times that suit family members and respect their needs serves to further empower the family and to increase the likelihood that they will be willing to engage in the treatment process.

There are some families of children with SED who appear to be unable to provide the level of care and nurturance needed by the child or adolescent. The argument in favor of working with children with SED in the context of their families may be best made by looking at these more difficult families and considering a clear alternative to home-based intervention: removal of children to an apparently more benign setting. Indeed, some youths with SED live in such severe psychosocial adversity that the first and ultimate intervention for them may be removal from their families. Placement away from the family may seem especially compelling at the start of a home-based intervention, when the full extent of the child's psychosocial adversity may become evident to his or her treatment team for the first time.

However, following the principle of the child's best interest, consideration of out-of-home placement must always be grounded in the presumption of the least detrimental alternative (Goldstein et al., 1996). This presumption suggests that each and every decision to make a change in a child's placement status contains potential risks as well as benefits. No choice is risk-free; risks and benefits coexist in the choice of no action, just as they do in the choice of placement in an institution. The presumption of the least detrimental alternative supports the use of interventions that are selected by careful assessment of each child and family. For maximum effectiveness, these interventions should be provided in the manner and place that represent the best fit for the child and are most likely to preserve his connections to those persons to whom he is most closely attached. In some cases, the least detrimental alternative may be to provide additional supports so that the child can continue to live with his or her family. In other cases, in which the family's functioning presents a more imminent risk to the child's safety and well-being, the least detrimental alternative may in fact involve foster or institution-based care. Whatever the decision, interest in the child's safety and well-being with all its attendant risks and benefits does not end when the decision to place has been made. Only when the child has a sense of permanency will he or she be able to move forward toward recovery.

### FIRST STEPS: ENTERING THE FAMILY ENVIRONMENT

When IICAPS clinicians cross the threshold into the world of the family, they are presented with a view into the most important domain in the child's microsystem. It is essential that IICAPS team members recognize that their presence in the home raises a myriad of questions and concerns. The team must communicate both verbally and by their actions the seriousness and importance of the IICAPS intervention and the reasons for their presence. From the outset the goals of all IICAPS interactions should be obvious, or at least explainable, to all involved.

Some family members may have their own beliefs about why unfamiliar people are coming to the home or what they will do while they are there. Family members may question the ways persons who may differ from them ethnically, culturally, economically, and/or educationally will view them. Others may be concerned about family integrity and worried that the identified child will be removed from the family system and placed in hospital. Some families with protective service histories may be concerned about possible reporting risks or how closely the family will be scrutinized. Team members, in turn, may have concerns about the conditions in the home that may affect their safety and may pose possible risks to their bodily integrity.

### Observation

Upon entering the home the IICAPS team is presented with a unique opportunity to glimpse the real world of the child and family. From this point forward the team is able to accumulate firsthand observations that will inform the treatment process. Working *in vivo* the team is able to view the complex, often unnoticed and unanticipated interactions that take place between children and the adults who care for them. From the time of their initial entrance into the complex, highly personal environment of the home, the team, with the assistance of the family, should be able to use their observations to piece together a narrative of the child's and family's history. This narrative can be considered the backbone of the intervention.

From the initial Phase of the work onward, team members are expected to be careful observers of the home environment and the activities that go on within it. It is particularly important to note the ways in which family members deal with the tasks and responsibilities of daily living and the manner in which they cope with crises and other stressful situations. Once within the child's world, the team assesses the family's relative stability and their willingness to change in the service of the child's recovery. As careful observers, team members can quickly gather a wealth of information about child and family functioning that might take months to compile in any other setting. The richness of these data greatly increases the authenticity of the treatment plan. This information grounds the work in the family's reality rather than in the fantasies of either the family or the treatment team.

### Fostering Engagement

Once inside the home, IICAPS teams are charged with engaging the child and family in the service of building the therapeutic alliance that is the basis of IICAPS treatment. Working directly in the home facilitates and supports the development of the alliance. Opportunities to engage authentically with families are available to the team from the initial stages of IICAPS intervention. The act of entering the home conveys the team's acceptance of the child and family and sets the stage for the establishment of a more nearly equal relationship. Once within the home, team members must remember that they are guests. They are not expected to assume any functions for the family; rather, their role is to act as a consultant to the family or as an agent on its behalf.

Although the team can be seen as powerful because it has knowledge that has not yet been communicated to the family, the family has control over the intervention. The family can choose to open the door to the team or turn them away by not answering their knock or leaving the home, sometimes ostensibly just to run an errand. The family can gather together for family sessions, or individual family members can busy themselves in other parts of the home with activities unrelated to the work of treatment. Family members can leave the room at will and not return. They can engage in the work or make it impossible to move forward. The behavior of family members will vary in accordance with the relationships that develop between them and the members of the team and their commitment to making the changes needed to assure the child's ability to remain safely in the home.

The antidote for behaviors that undermine treatment lies primarily in the team's ability to convey acceptance, mutual trust, and respect. In this context, acceptance should be construed as the team's willingness to involve the child and family as full partners in the work of treatment. Trust emerges from interactions between the team and the family that are dependable, reliable, and transparent. Respect is communicated to the family through the professionalism of the team members in all aspects of their interactions with the family, such as their demeanor while in the home and community, their language, their dress, and their commitment to steadfast, timely maintenance of their scheduled appointments. Having realistic expectations helps the team to work with resistant or distrustful families. Helping families to set achievable goals that can be attained through small, incremental advances often gives families the confidence to move forward in treatment and deepens the working alliance.

All IICAPS services are voluntary. Although families must agree to an in-home intervention before a referral is made to an IICAPS program, some families are more willing than others to engage actively with the team. It is not unusual for families to test the commitment and acceptance of the team by disregarding the treatment plan, failing to keep appointments, or scheduling competing activities for the child. Through supervision and training, team members are helped to recognize the meaning of these behaviors and find ways to work through the issues that could potentially derail the treatment process.

### Creating a Therapeutic Space

As we have described, the initial task of the IICAPS team is to foster the child's and family's engagement in the treatment through the development of a therapeutic alliance. Therefore, it is essential that the intervention begin honestly with a clear statement of purpose. At their first meeting, team members are expected to introduce themselves to the child and family and explain the reason they have been referred for IICAPS services. They then describe the process by which they will work in partnership with the family to set the goals of the intervention.

As quickly as possible, the family and the IICAPS team establish a mutual understanding of why the team is joining with the family. In the first session the team and the family lay out a plan for dealing with emergency situations should they arise. They also address any practical barriers to treatment such as lack of access to a telephone or an impending eviction. The team then attempts to establish clear expectations for treatment by developing specific goals and action steps that will lead to the desired outcomes of reduced risk of hospitalization and improvement in the child's symptomology.

The ability to provide psychiatric treatment in the home depends upon the ability of the family and the team to establish clear therapeutic and spatial boundaries. Treatment cannot take place if members of the family do not feel safe while they are engaged in the process. Working with the team, the family identifies the physical space that will permit confidential exchanges, and clarifies the lines of authority and channels of communication that are necessary elements of the intervention. As preparation for treatment moves forward, the real work of IICAPS is ready to begin.

## THE USE OF THERAPEUTIC TECHNIQUES

Three therapeutic techniques are useful throughout the IICAPS treatment: reframing, therapeutic anticipation, and expansion of the therapeutic surface. *Reframing* consists of recasting self-defeating statements and ideas into constructs that allow for healthy growth. For reframing to have a chance to be useful it must embrace the reality of family members' perceptions while at the same time offering a new view of the world. *Therapeutic anticipation* is the technique of explicitly describing all aspects of the IICAPS intervention and preparing family members for the next step in treatment. Therapeutic anticipation is intended to decrease the ambiguity of purpose and to increase the structure of interaction. By these mechanisms therapeutic anticipation tends to allay anxiety in family members and create a set of expected interactions that provide a framework for assessment. Paraphrasing advice for effective public speaking, therapeutic anticipation means "say what you're suggesting to do together, then do it together, then end by describing what you just have accomplished together." *Expansion of the therapeutic surface* is a technique that begins with the presumption that the work of treatment can occur only in areas related to the issues that have been acknowledged openly by the family and thus are available for authentic discussion. Such issues are considered to be "on the therapeutic surface." Quite frequently, powerful, unpleasant emotions like fear, shame, or anger prevent such authentic discussions. When authentic discussion is blocked it is difficult for therapeutic process to occur. When this situation arises, team members should strategize together about the ways in which they can unblock the discussion and expand the therapeutic surface. The first step in this process is finding a way to reframe the taboo subject so that it is less infused with intolerable emotion. The next step is linking the previously taboo subject with the problem to be solved.

Specifically, the treatment team, with the help of supervision, identifies those factors that are deemed important for therapeutic progress but are not yet able to be acknowledged authentically in discussions with the child and family members. The endpoint of the process of expanding the therapeutic surface is marked by the creation of specific elements of the treatment plan that address the issues that were important issues within the family but were previously unable to be addressed openly.

The basic clinical skills required to treat children and families with severe psychological disturbances effectively are not site dependent. However, delivering psychiatric services in the home provides opportunities to influence family functioning that may not be as readily available in other settings. By accepting the reality of the child's and family's world and working to support the attainment of their own goals, IICAPS interventions can help families to achieve higher levels of self-efficacy and competence. By actually entering into the life of the family, IICAPS is better able to enhance the family's sense of control over the environment and increase the ability of family members to function adaptively.

# Chapter 4 Home-Based Work
# the IICAPS Way

IICAPS embraces the general precepts of home-based treatment as the starting point of the intervention. The IICAPS model strives to provide enough structure that the treatment of each SED youth and each component of his/her treatment is measurable while still permitting the flexibility and creativity that are essential ingredients of this work. If the model is structured inadequately, evaluation is not possible at any level. Too much structure will compromise the ability of the model to address the complex problems that characterize SED youths and their families.

IICAPS treatment is conceptualized as a two-dimensional matrix. One dimension consists of the specific treatments or interventions that are utilized to achieve specific treatment goals. These specific treatments may be selected from the array of evidence-based or best practices that are currently available. These treatment modalities may have their own structure as prescribed in a treatment manual or by treatment guidelines. Other interventions may incorporate techniques, tools, and activities that reflect the combined clinical experience and expertise of team members and supervisors. Team members are expected to be familiar with and make use of a wide range of treatment options that are selected as appropriate to meet the individual needs of the child and family.

The second dimension of IICAPS treatment is defined by IICAPS Fidelity Mechanisms, especially those used to measure fidelity to the model at the case level. These mechanisms provide and reinforce the overall structure that facilitates and organizes the implementation of specific treatments. These structures assure fidelity to the IICAPS model by providing specific guidelines that are designed to promote ongoing engagement and effective problem solving. Without these structures, maintenance of both the therapeutic alliance and treatment focus will likely be compromised. The team and family members alike are at risk of becoming lost in the morass of interconnected clinical problems. The IICAPS treatment structures and Fidelity Mechanisms at the case, clinician, program, and network levels are intended to facilitate, evaluate, and refine the work in a consistent and continuous fashion. The four levels of structures move from direct-level treatment delivery (case level) to more general clinical administration (network level). Each level depends on the next level for definition and context.

## IICAPS CASE-LEVEL FIDELITY MECHANISMS

IICAPS case-level Fidelity Mechanisms consist of three nested structural types: *Principles, Concepts,* and *Tools.* These mechanisms guide the implementation of IICAPS treatment with each child and family and allow for the measurement of adherence to the IICAPS model. Because of the role they play in guiding the treatment process, the case-level Fidelity Mechanisms are the most fundamental components of the IICAPS approach. The Principles, Concepts, and Tools that characterize IICAPS and provide its structure are nested in a manner that is analogous to the nesting of the four levels of Fidelity Mechanisms. Each structural element is dependent on the preceeding structure for definition and context.

### Principles

Co-Construction, Transparency, Practicality, Immediacy, and Adherence to IICAPS Concepts are the five overarching IICAPS Principles. *Co-Construction,* the first IICAPS Principle, requires that the child, the family, and the IICAPS team mutually agree on all elements of the treatment. The Treatment Plan itself must reflect the needs, aims, and beliefs as they are expressed by the family and as they relate to the child's recovery. It is essential that all treatment elements are consistent with the language and the culture of the family. Authentic and open communication between the child, the family, and the team enables the process of Co-Construction to maximize the therapeutic potential of each treatment element. Family members should ask the question "Is this my goal that I want to work on now?"

*Transparency* advocates that every component of the treatment process be understandable and reasonable to everyone involved in the treatment. Unfortunately, most mental health treatments are so filled with jargon and unexplained assumptions that the vast majority of people receiving these treatments, and perhaps implementing them, do so on faith rather than understanding. Transparency is crucial to a treatment approach that requires ongoing partnership with youths and family members. The issue of transparency, or the lack thereof, arises at the very start of any home-based treatment and generally continues until past the end of treatment. The child and family members usually wonder, "Why are these people here in my home? What are their motivations? What do they want from me? Can I tell them I mistrust them?" Similar important questions continue throughout treatment and beyond; family members may ask themselves, "What did we accomplish? Are we supposed to keep working on this? Why did we end when we did?" Transparency does not apply only to youths with SED and the members of their families. Clinicians may wonder why certain parts of the treatment plan were developed or why certain steps are supposed to occur in treatment. Both asking and answering all of these and many other questions are crucial for the work to progress. Some questions will be answered by the name of the structure itself, thus freeing up time and energy for other questions. For example, the components of IICAPS treatment are named in standard English rather than in a special IICAPS language. The Principle of Transparency extends to the IICAPS model itself, in which there is nothing hidden.

*Practicality,* the third IICAPS Principle, states that each person involved in IICAPS treatment should be asked to do only those activities that are achievable and reasonable for that person. All too often, behavioral health interventions make incorrect assumptions or have unrealistic expectations of children, family members, and clinicians. Such incorrect assumptions can lead to the failure of the treatment effort. While any failure can be discouraging, failure based upon inaccurate assumptions of capability frequently results in blaming, which in turn can poison the entire treatment alliance. The Principle of Practicality dictates that the IICAPS team and the family members ascertain whether a particular person has the skill set to undertake a particular task by asking, "Do I have the skills and knowledge to accomplish this goal?" If the person cannot reasonably accomplish the task with the current skill set, then the task must be modified or dropped or the person must be provided the missing skills before the desired task is attempted.

*Immediacy,* the fourth IICAPS Principle, advocates that interventions be practiced on a regular (daily, or at least weekly) basis in order to accomplish treatment goals in the present and near future. This Principle actually has two components: (1) there is an expectation that tasks must be worked on frequently (that is, daily); (2) the focus of work is on the present or near future. Family members must ask, "Am I working on this goal daily or at least weekly?" The Principle of Immediacy reminds all participants in IICAPS interventions that change in long-established patterns requires sustained effort on a regular basis. In addition, only work that is focused on the present can be measured in the present. Such measurement and refinement in the present are requirements for any sustained progress toward goals.

*Adherence to IICAPS Concepts,* the fifth IICAPS Principle, emphasizes the importance of employing the basic, case-level constructs in the implementation of IICAPS treatment. Adherence to the model is mediated and measured via Principles, Concepts, and Tools. Adherence to the IICAPS model provides all participants with a critically important road map that permits the evaluation of individual case effectiveness as well as the effectiveness of the IICAPS model itself at team, program, and network levels. At the case level, each participant should assess at regular intervals both clinical progress and the degree of adherence to the model. If there is both a lack of progress and a lack of adherence, then the first task is to modify the work so that greater adherence to the model becomes more likely. At the team, program, and network levels, effectiveness of the IICAPS model can be evaluated by analyzing the relationship between clinical outcomes and adherence to the model's structure, specifically the implementation and use of IICAPS Principles, Concepts, and Tools.

### Concepts

The IICAPS Concepts are the basic ideational elements of each IICAPS treatment. They are presented in the order in which the clinical team explores them with the child and family members. IICAPS Concepts form the basis for IICAPS Tools, which not only guide the intervention but also serve as the final structure for measuring fidelity to the model.

The *Main Problem* is the behavior, described in the words of the family members, that puts the child at significant risk for requiring institution-based treatment.

*Strengths & Vulnerabilities* are those factors, behaviors, interactions, conditions, and beliefs, described in the words of the family members, which affect the Main Problem directly or indirectly. Strengths keep the Main Problem from getting worse; Vulnerabilities keep the Main Problem from getting better. The team works with the family to identify the Strengths & Vulnerabilities in each Domain that appear to influence the Main Problem, and act either as barriers to or promoters of the child's behavior. Identification of Strengths & Vulnerabilities is influenced by factors described by developmental psychopathology as being important to the course of the child's developmental trajectory.

IICAPS treatment identifies Strengths & Vulnerabilities in four *Domains:*

- Child Domain (interaction of child and his internal resources)
  attachments and attachment quality
  self-representations
  coping mechanisms
  temperament styles
  mental health and physical health
- Family Domain (interaction of child, his parents, and other family members)
  co-parenting styles
  parental and sibling relationships
  conflict resolution skills
  level of family functioning
  boundaries
  limit setting
  discipline style
- School Domain (interaction of child and school environment)
  appropriateness of school placement
  child's ability to learn in the current setting
  flexibility of school personnel
  ability of school personnel to understand the child and to work collaboratively
    with the family, the child, and the IICAPS team
- Environment and Other Systems Domain (interaction of child with other services
    and systems)
  adequacy of housing
  neighborhood safety
  spiritual and recreational resources
  community supports
  access to mental health, legal, health, and juvenile justice systems and the like

Three *Phases* demarcate specific treatment epochs and utilize Phase-specific tasks. The Phases are overlapping in the sense that the tasks of one

Phase lead to the work of the tasks in the next Phase. Thus, the final task in the first Phase creates the plan for the middle Phase, and the final task in the middle Phase creates the plan for the last Phase. Each of the three consecutive Phases of treatment identifies and addresses factors in each of the four Domains. Although the Phases are distinct and are operationally defined, considerable blurring can occur among them. When progress is blocked in the middle Phase, the team and family members may need to return to the first Phase in the process of treatment refinement. For this reason the divisions of Phases serve as guidelines, not as concrete boundaries.

The three Phases of IICAPS treatment, which are accomplished by the joint efforts of the treatment team, the child and the family members, are:

- Assessment & Engagement
- Work & Action
- Ending & Wrap-Up

The Assessment & Engagement Phase begins with the creation of a plan for addressing child and family emergencies and ends with the development of the Treatment Plan. The Treatment Plan has Goals and specific Action Steps in each of the four Domains. An Attainment Scale accompanies each Goal and its attendant Action Steps. Work & Action, the middle Phase, is the period when the Action Steps connected with each Goal in the Treatment Plan are expected to be implemented. The Treatment Plan is reviewed every 6 weeks by the IICAPS team and the family members using the Attainment Scales to rate the progress on each Goal and Action Step. If the Attainment Scales indicate that treatment is not progressing in an adequate fashion, the IICAPS clinical team and the family members systematically refine the Treatment Plan. The Work & Action Phase ends when enough Goals have been reached that the clinical team and the family members agree that the child is at greatly reduced risk for institutional treatment. The final step of this Phase is the creation of the Ending & Wrap-Up Plan, the description of the Action Steps that need to be accomplished in each Domain so that the child and family are linked to any and all services necessary to insure continued improved functioning. The Ending & Wrap-Up Plan is a mutual creation of the treatment team, child, and family members.

Ending & Wrap-Up, the final Phase of IICAPS treatment, is guided by the implementation of the Ending & Wrap-Up Plan. It ends when enough of the Action Steps of the Ending & Wrap-Up Plan have been accomplished and there is a reasonable probability that the gains made in IICAPS treatment will be maintained. The final step of the Ending & Wrap-Up Phase is the creation, with the child and family members, of the Treatment Summary & Discharge Recommendation Plan. This document describes the original reasons for referral to IICAPS, the course of treatment, and the various activities and services that the child and family will continue to use after the end of IICAPS treatment. The joint creation of this summary of IICAPS work and the agreed-upon recommendations for work after IICAPS is designed to help facilitate the continuation of the health-promoting process.

### Tools

IICAPS *Tools* serve as guides to IICAPS interventions and as Fidelity Mechanisms. Tools outline specific tasks that require the joint effort of the team and family members with the aim of creating a specific document for a specific purpose at a specific step in a specific *Phase* of treatment. Tools assist simultaneously in engagement, assessment, intervention, supervision, and quality assurance.

Each Tool enhances the therapeutic relationship by increasing the experience of empathy and providing the information needed to inform treatment. The use of the Tools is a therapeutic experience for the child and family and enables all elements of the specific treatment process to be transparent to the child and family, clinical team, and supervisor. This "4-in-1" aspect of each Tool informs its use. A Tool is never simply "paperwork" to be completed for the sake of a chart audit. Tools enhance engagement and serve to structure activities between the IICAPS team and family members. These activities are opportunities for reframing, therapeutic anticipation, and especially expansion of the therapeutic surface. Importantly, Tools provide a framework with which to measure treatment progress. Tools allow the IICAPS team and family members to ask and to answer the question "How are we doing in our work together?" Each IICAPS Tool is described in relation to each of the three phases of treatment.

THE TOOLS FOR ENGAGEMENT &
ASSESSMENT PHASE

*Immediate Action Plan.* Beginning at the time of initial referral and continuing until the end of treatment, the clinical team and the family should become proficient at evaluating and addressing issues on two parallel but different intervals of time. One interval, devoted to the development of the IICAPS Treatment Plan, usually unfolds over a period of weeks. The second interval, that of the development and implementation of the Immediate Action Plan, generally occurs over hours and days. The Immediate Action Plan addresses issues that require intervention in the very short term. Typically such issues are related either to imminent danger or to pressing needs of the family for basic functioning. Identifying these issues and implementing a plan to address them immediately are crucial for child safety as well as for the development of a therapeutic alliance with the child and the family. The challenge for the family, the treatment team, and the IICAPS supervisor is to separate those issues that actually require an Immediate Action Plan from issues that should be addressed through the more formal treatment planning process. Overlooking issues that require an Immediate Action Plan may create risk of injury and/or alienation of the family. Conversely, including nonemergent issues in the Immediate Action Plan may threaten to shift the IICAPS intervention into a crisis-driven rather than a longer-term planning process. At minimum, every case should have an Immediate Action Plan that specifies who, when, why, and how the IICAPS team should be contacted should an emergency arise.

In many cases the creation of the Immediate Action Plan can be left as a relatively informal process. This process might include the clinical team's providing the child and family with written information about under what circumstances and by what mechanisms the clinical team is to be contacted for emergencies, changes in appointments, and other pressing matters. In addition, the clinical team with the child and family outlines the several specific tasks to be accomplished in the first few weeks of treatment that are necessary for work to proceed in a safe, productive fashion. Examples of such tasks are obtaining telephone service, prepaid calling cards, transportation vouchers, or emergency fuel and removing firearms from the household. The contents of the Immediate Action Plan must be presented in supervision and included in the child's chart.

If the team and supervisor are concerned that progress is stalled in the Assessment & Engagement Phase, they should create a more formal Immediate Action Plan. The plan should use the following format: (1) specify the Action Steps that should be taken in relation to the child's safety and/or fulfillment of basic needs and (2) create an Attainment Scale for each Action Step.

*Defining the Main Problem.* The Main Problem is the behavior, usually involving danger to self or others, that creates most of the risk that the child will require institutional treatment. The Main Problem must always be defined in the language of the family members. Frequently the Main Problem is closely related to the reason for referral but may not be identical with it. While specification of the Main Problem may appear self-evident to the clinical team, developing consensus with the child and the members of his family about the specific behavior that threatens his ability to remain safely at home is crucial to the engagement process and essential to the development of the list of Strengths & Vulnerabilities that are related to the Main Problem. Not infrequently both the clinical team and family members may feel that defining the Main Problem by describing one of the child's behaviors is excessively reductionistic and may be misleading. After all, the youth and family members have complicated lives in which many problems are interconnected. However, it is important to define a Main Problem in this narrow fashion because of, not in spite of, the complexity of problems. Treatment that is not anchored by a specific focal point is in danger of drifting. Such treatment drift risks loss of effectiveness.

Defining the Main Problem is the anchor for IICAPS treatment. The Main Problem, stated in the words of the family members, is the primary problem, the *raison d'être*, to be addressed by them in their work with the IICAPS team. The Main Problem should be a statement of vulnerability, the behavior or problem about which the youth and parents are most worried. An important reason for effective work to falter is that the Main Problem loses its motivating meaning. The IICAPS approach of problem identification and problem solving, treatment planning, and treatment implementation can be visualized as an hourglass-shaped phenomenon. The initial Assessment & Engagement Phase casts a broad net for information and relationship building, represented by the top half of the hourglass. The information gathered during this phase is used to refine the Main Problem, which becomes the focus of the work, the narrow point between the top and bottom of the hourglass. Progressing further, the creation of a Treatment Plan and its actual implementation are represented by the broadening of the lower half of the hourglass.

IICAPS teams develop and use a 10-point Severity Scale to maintain the family's focus on the Main Problem. This Scale provides a metric for the family and team members to periodically rate the likelihood that the Main Problem will require the youth's hospitalization immediately or in the very near future.

*The Genogram.* The *Genogram,* another IICAPS Tool, is a standard family assessment device with well-described symbols and procedures (McGoldrick, Gerson, and Shellenberger, 1999). The drawing of a three-generational

Genogram with the family provides a unique picture of family members, current household membership, significant changes in permanency arrangements for the identified patient and other important life events, and the emotional relationships among family members and other significant people. Although all the information displayed in the Genogram is provided by family members, the process of producing the Genogram may reveal aspects of intergenerational patterns of behavior, family relationships, and physical and mental health status that have not been acknowledged previously. This information expands the therapeutic surface and informs the treatment process.

Children who have experienced significant changes in placement need to have several Genograms, each labeled by dates in the child's life. Like all other IICAPS Tools, the Genogram is designed to promote four critical processes simultaneously: engagement, assessment, intervention, and quality assurance/supervision.

In order to accomplish the first three processes, all members of the child's immediate family should be involved in the creation of the Genogram. A copy of the three-generation Genogram should be left with them when it is completed. From time to time some family members provide data that other family members consider too sensitive to be placed on the genogram for all to see. The clinical team must follow the lead of those who object to the disclosure of this information by including only those data that are acceptable to everyone. However, omissions from the Genogram must be viewed as important clinical data that, though not yet available to be acknowledged authentically by the family, will eventually need to be addressed.

*Inventory of Strengths & Vulnerabilities. The Inventory of Strengths & Vulnerabilities* in four Domains is a catalogue, in the language of the family, of the relevant Strengths & Vulnerabilities that directly or indirectly maintain the Main Problem at its current level of intensity/severity *and* can be influenced by the IICAPS intervention. When developing the inventory of Strengths & Vulnerabilities in the four Domains, the team and family should examine the child's entire microsystem. The team and family members then ask whether and how the identified Strengths & Vulnerabilities are related to the Main Problem. While many Strengths and Vulnerabilities may be considered, if a particular factor has no connection, either direct or indirect, to the Main Problem, it should be dropped from the active working inventory. When the connection of the identified factors with the maintenance of the Main Problem is supported by data from developmental psychopathology, it is the most convincing.

Similar to the specification of the Main Problem, the inventory of Strengths & Vulnerabilities in the four Domains should be the result of building consensus with the family. This process is crucial to the engagement process and prepares the family for the next step, the development of the Eco-Domain Map.

*The Eco-Domain Map. The Eco-Domain Map* is a graphic depiction of the initial working hypotheses related to the ways in which the identified Strengths & Vulnerabilities in the four Domains maintain the Main Problem's current levels of severity and intensity. In the Eco-Domain Map, the Main Problem is written in a rectangle in the middle of the page; Strengths are placed inside triangles to convey that they are fulcrums for goal attainment; Vulnerabilities are placed inside ovals to convey that these are obstacles to progress; health-promoting interactions are depicted by double-lined arrows, and illness-promoting interactions with single-lined arrows. The choices of Main Problem, the Strengths & Vulnerabilities that maintain it, the direction and valence of the interactions, the various connections, and the proximity of the supporting factors to the Main Problem should all be consistent with concepts and data from developmental psychopathology.

The team and family members populate the Eco-Domain Map in layered fashion, beginning with the Main Problem and then with Child, Family, School, and finally with Environment and Other System Domain elements, in that order (see Figures 4.1 a–d). When adding elements of a particular Domain, the team members start with the most obviously important Vulnerabilities and add the Strengths that are likely to mitigate or counterbalance these Vulnerabilities. The team and family members should understand that the process of creating the Eco-Domain Map is as important as the finished product, since this process provides a vehicle for the first holistic and dynamic understanding of the factors that maintain the Main Problem. The Eco-Domain Map must have a high degree of congruence with the inventory of Strengths & Vulnerabilities in the four Domains. Since the Eco-Domain Map is viewed as an evolving hypothesis, it is always a work in progress. The Eco-Domain Map is a collaborative effort involving the family, treatment team, supervisor, and members of rounds. The first draft of the Eco-Domain Map should be simple, involving the fewest possible factors (Strengths & Vulnerabilities) needed to ameliorate the Main Problem; successive drafts may become more complex, reflecting the increase in clinical understanding by the team and family. The Eco-Domain Map is the basis of the Treatment Plan; therefore the Eco-Domain Map and the Treatment Plan should always be concordant.

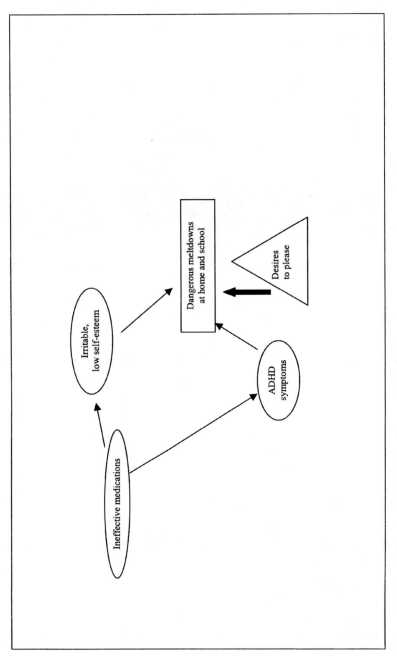

Figure 4.1a. Eco-Domain Map: Main Problem and Child

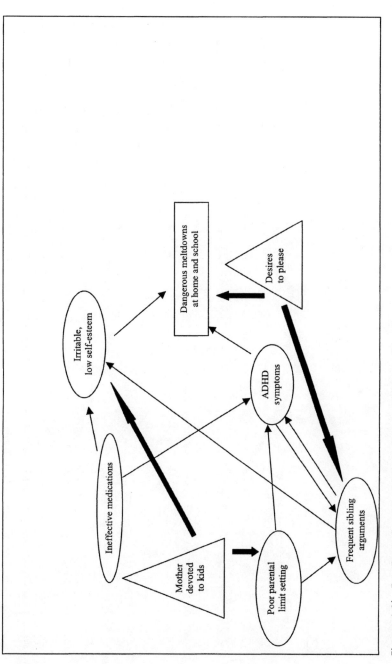

Figure 4.1b. Eco-Domain Map: Main Problem, Child, and Family

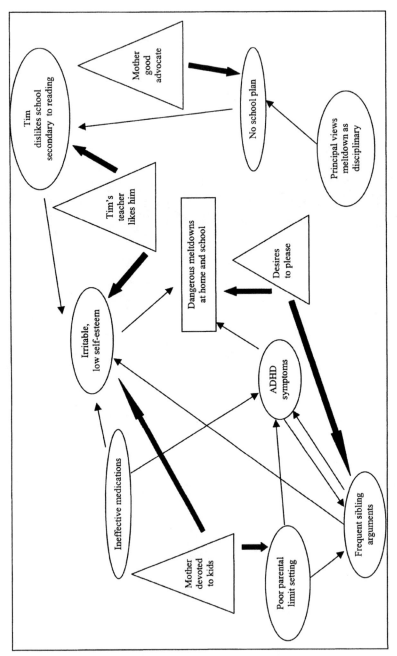

Figure 4.1c. Eco-Domain Map: Main Problem, Child, Family, and School

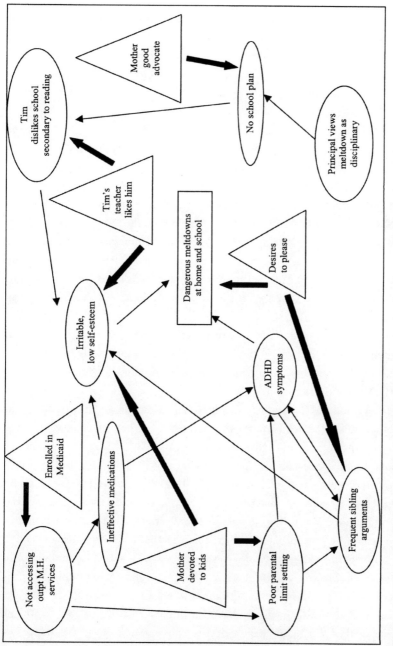

Figure 4.1d. Eco-Domain Map: Main Problem, Child, Family, Physical Environment and Other Systems

*The Treatment Plan.* The *Treatment Plan* is the last IICAPS Tool developed in the Assessment & Engagement Phase. The process of developing the Treatment Plan is an iterative, collaborative process that flows directly from the preceding steps of specification of the Main Problem, creating the inventory of Strengths & Vulnerabilities in four Domains, and drawing the Eco-Domain Map. The Treatment Plan consists of Goals stated in the family's words, Action Steps in the family's words, and a corresponding 10-point Attainment Scale for each Goal and Action Step.

The Treatment Plan has Goals and attendant Action Steps in each of the four Domains: Child, Family, School, and Environment and Other Systems. As indicated above, the first version of the Treatment Plan should err on the side of simplicity rather than comprehensiveness. In accordance with this guideline, this first version should have no more than two Goals in each Domain. The Treatment Plan must be consistent with the five IICAPS Principles of Co-Construction, Transparency, Practicality, Immediacy, and Adherence to the IICAPS Constructs. After each Goal is chosen, the team and family members identify specific Action Steps to accomplish the Goal. To remain consistent with the IICAPS Principles, these Action Steps should be clearly related to ameliorating the Main Problem, developed mutually by the family members and the team (Co-Construction), understandable and reasonable to everyone (Transparency), able to be implemented by the family members and the team (Practicality), and requiring regular, usually daily or weekly, work by family members (Immediacy).

In addition the Goals and Action Steps should be consistent with the causal mechanisms described by developmental psychopathology as relevant to the maintenance of the child's disturbance. Each Goal and Action Step must be connected to specific interactions of Strengths, Vulnerabilities, and the Main Problem on the Eco-Domain Map. The IICAPS team and family must be able to move from each element of the Treatment Plan to specific parts of the Eco-Domain Map so that the relationship between the Treatment Plan and the sustaining process depicted by the Eco-Domain Map is transparent.

A 10-point Attainment Scale accompanies each Goal and Action Step. The Attainment Scales are most effective if specific behavioral examples are provided for at least the lowest and highest levels. Every six weeks the IICAPS team and family members evaluate the implementation of the Treatment Plan together. The main purpose of this regular assessment is to enhance engagement and provide a basis for ongoing refinement of the Treatment Plan. Therefore the process of using the Attainment Scales is at least as important as the actual values assigned to them. For this reason, disagreements between the clinical team and family members about specific ratings must be viewed as opportunities for more authentic engagement in the treatment process rather than as obstacles to progress. One approach to recording such disagreements is simply to place the rater's initials next to each rating on a particular scale rather than to insist on complete consensus.

Creation of the first draft of the Treatment Plan marks the end of the Assessment & Engagement Phase and the beginning of the Work & Action Phase. Usually the treatment team and family have been working together for several weeks before this draft of the Treatment Plan is completed and ready for implementation. Typically, some Goals have already been identified by the family members and the team, and despite the delay between the first visit and the completion of the Treatment Plan, initial work on these Goals has begun. Nonetheless, it is essential that these early goals be included in the more formal Treatment Plan.

The development of the IICAPS Treatment Plan, including Goals, Action Steps, and Attainment Scales, is both a goal in itself and an opportunity to engage the family in a specific and explicit discussion geared toward problem solving. The development of the Treatment Plan is also a key tool in the process of engaging the family as full partners in the treatment.

TOOLS FOR THE WORK & ACTION PHASE

*Treatment Plan Refinement Process.* The *Treatment Plan Refinement Process* is an explicit approach to improving the implementation of the Treatment Plan in response to actual experiences of the family and the team. The first step in the Treatment Plan Refinement Process is the evaluation of the progress of treatment. This evaluation, guided by the rating of the Attainment Scales, is completed every six weeks as a joint effort of the treatment team, the child, and family members. The data based upon the evaluation are presented in alternate rounds during the Work & Action Phase. If there is an indication of lack of progress toward Goal Attainment or failure to implement the planned Action Steps, the IICAPS team, and the child and family should discuss the reasons why the treatment process is stalled and develop a strategy to address the problems.

Regular assessment of Action Step implementation and of progress toward Goal Attainment is absolutely essential in order to avoid becoming mired in an ineffective treatment alliance. An ineffective treatment alliance is characterized by the appearance of agreement about treatment without any of the significant work of treatment occurring and presents a major obstacle to reducing the severity of the Main Problem. An ineffective treatment alliance wastes the precious resources represented by the time and energy of everyone involved in an IICAPS intervention. The regular use of the Attainment Scales to evaluate treatment progress follows the IICAPS Principles of Transparency and Practicality and assures that the Goals and Action Steps are understood and constructed in such a way that each member of the team and family is capable of implementing each component of the plan.

In the process of evaluating the Treatment Plan the team and family members may observe a lack of progress characterized by one or more of the following: (1) Action Steps are not being implemented, (2) Goals are not being accomplished, and (3) the Main Problem is getting worse. Often when the progress of treatment is stalled the reason is that the child and other family members feel that the Goals and the Action Steps fail to realistically reflect their needs and abilities. In some cases the child and family, in an effort to please the IICAPS team, may have acquiesced to Goals that they believed represented the wishes of the team members. In other cases the child and family were not yet ready to engage in an authentic manner. At times the Goals and the Action Steps may not be consistent with the Principle of Practicality because they are not congruent with the capacities of the child and family members and are too ambitious to be achieved.

More specifically, in the evaluation of the Treatment Plan, specific Goal and Action Step attainments are compared with those Goals that were previously desired and agreed upon. Comparisons between actual and desired progress are rated by predefined Attainment Scales, and the Treatment Plan is refined when there is a significant discrepancy between the desired and actual achievement of Goals and implementation of Action Steps. Lack of progress indicates that the entire process of the Treatment Plan development and implementation needs to be reviewed. After the team and family members complete this systematic review, new or modified Goals and Action Steps are developed that are more likely to be successful. The IICAPS Treatment Refinement Process is structured by the sequential use of the specific IICAPS Tools.

The IICAPS Treatment Plan Refinement Process provides data that can be used by supervisors to support the clinical team. In turn, the team should encourage family members to engage in hypothesis testing about the causes and correlates of particular problems within the family and the reasons that desired improvements have not occurred. All members of the IICAPS

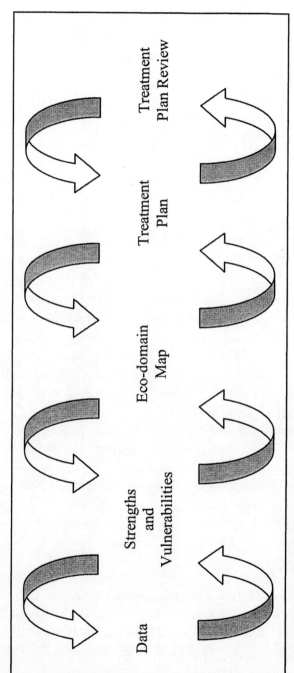

Data

Strengths
and
Vulnerabilities

Eco-domain
Map

Treatment
Plan

Treatment
Plan Review

Figure 4.2. Treatment Refinement Process

intervention use the IICAPS Treatment Plan Refinement Process as a template for reevaluation of the Treatment Plan. The team and the appropriate family members should systematically review all the steps of the IICAPS process leading to the Treatment Plan as depicted in Figure 4.2. Usually the three most important questions to review are:

- Does the Eco-Domain Map accurately depict the processes that sustain the Main Problem?
- Does the Treatment Plan reflect the processes identified by the Eco-Domain Map in each of the four Domains?
- Does the Treatment Plan have achievable Goals and Action Steps that change the sustaining process depicted on the Eco-Domain Map?

TOOLS FOR ENDING & WRAP-UP PHASE

*Ending & Wrap-Up Plan.* The final IICAPS Tool to be developed in the Work & Action Phase is the *Ending & Wrap-Up Plan.* The team, child, and family create the Ending & Wrap-Up Plan when sufficient progress has been made toward accomplishing the Goals of the Treatment Plan and together they have deemed that the child's risk of requiring institutional treatment is significantly reduced. The Ending & Wrap-Up Plan is a list of Action Steps in each Domain that are needed to maintain all the child and family Goals that have been accomplished during the Work & Action Phase. This list of Action Steps is accompanied by a 10-point Attainment Scale that provides an individualized metric for measuring progress.

The IICAPS team, child, and family use the Ending & Wrap-Up Plan to guide the work in this phase of treatment. The phase-specific Attainment Scale, which is completed by the team, child and family, provides a vehicle by which they, the supervisors, and rounds attendees can systematically review case progress. In addition to providing structure for the ending phase of treatment, the Ending & Wrap-Up Plan is a concrete but gentle way to introduce the process of saying good-bye, with all the feelings and behaviors that such a process may elicit.

*The Treatment Summary & Discharge Recommendations.* This is the last Tool to be developed in the Ending & Wrap-Up Phase. The Treatment Summary & Discharge Recommendations document describes the course of treatment as well as the mutually agreed-upon recommendations for the child and family following the end of the IICAPS intervention. This document, like all IICAPS Tools, is co-constructed by family members and the

IICAPS treatment team. After they create the first draft, it is reviewed by the supervisor, presented in rounds, and then brought back to the child and family for comments and final editing. After appropriate changes are made, IICAPS treatment team members, child, and parents sign the Treatment Summary & Discharge Recommendation. The family members are provided with one or more copies; one copy is placed in the IICAPS chart.

# Chapter 5 Specifics of
# IICAPS Treatment

While each child and family receiving IICAPS services is unique, the majority of IICAPS families share a number of characteristics in the four targeted Domains. Among the issues that emerge frequently in the process of creating IICAPS Treatment Plans are the following:

- The identified child is experiencing an inadequately treated psychiatric disorder that has resulted in specific emotional and behavioral disturbances that place the child at risk for requiring institution-based treatment.
- Family functioning is likely to be marked by ineffective limit setting, household disorganization, and difficulty providing appropriate parenting such as effective limit setting and emotional support.
- School programming may be inadequate to meet the child's special educational needs.
- Linkage to and utilization of social, financial, medical, behavioral health, spiritual, housing, and recreational resources are inadequate to meet the child and family's needs.

IICAPS treatment planning reflects the assessment of these common characteristics in the context of developmental psychopathology and assures that the four Domain-related elements will be addressed in each child's Treatment Plan.

An important question for the IICAPS team and the family members asks which of the specific treatments should be provided by the team members directly and which should be provided by other community resources. On one hand, direct provision of services by team members has several advantages, including enhancing engagement, reinforcing the IICAPS model, and increasing the likelihood of implementation of those treatments. On the other hand, having other treaters provide specific treatments such as clinic-based services during the IICAPS intervention may have its own advantages. Since IICAPS is a time-limited intervention, having the family members receive services from clinic-based providers before IICAPS is finished increases the likelihood of service continuity beyond the duration of the intervention. Some children and family members may begin the IICAPS intervention with their own clinic-based services in place. If the relevant family members are satisfied with these services, the IICAPS team must work with the family to develop a plan to insure maximum collaboration with these clinic-based providers. In addition to their ability to offer long-term continuity of care, clinic-based providers may have special expertise in a needed treatment that is outside the skill set of the IICAPS team. Finally, engaging the family members in needed clinic-based services empowers them to access those resources in a more typical and sustainable fashion.

## CHILD DOMAIN

Direct psychiatric treatment of SED youth, as specified in the Child Domain of the Treatment Plan, generally falls into two categories: pharmacotherapy and psychosocial treatments. Although psychopharmacotherapy for SED youth is still in its rudimentary stages of development, a few medications have been shown to be dramatically effective. Many more have supporting evidence for usefulness in the amelioration of problematic psychiatric symptoms. Effective psychopharmacotherapy requires several components: a judicious psychiatric evaluation, an effective therapeutic alliance, ongoing assessment of main effect and side effects of medications, and adherence to the dosing regimen. IICAPS treatment brings all of these elements of psychopharmacotherapy to the treatment of each child and family. The Treatment Plan may specify who will perform the initial and ongoing psychiatric assessment, what medications are to be taken when and for what, and how the child and family members will follow the prescribed medication regimen.

The other primary treatment category for youth with SED is comprised of specific psychosocial treatment modalities such as social skills training, problem-solving training, anger management training, and cognitive-behavioral therapies for depression, anxiety, and trauma (Kazdin and Weisz, 1998; Chambless and Ollendick, 2001). These treatments may be provided by one or both members of the IICAPS team, or by a community provider who is collaborating with the overall IICAPS treatment effort. Regardless of the provider, the necessary details of the treatment (who, what, when) are specified in the Treatment Plan.

## FAMILY DOMAIN

Elements of the Treatment Plan in the Family Domain generally focus on improving the family's ability to solve problems and to meet the developmental needs of family members, especially as related to limit setting and the support of appropriate generational boundaries and roles. These goals may be accomplished by using elements of problem-solving training (D'Zurilla and Nezu, 1999), parent management training (Kazdin, 2005), and functional family therapy (Alexander et al., 2000). Regardless of the therapeutic technique, the Treatment Plan must specify what tasks (Action Steps) each family member will be undertaking in the service of achieving better family functioning. Specific family-based therapeutic approaches may be used by the IICAPS team members and/or by another therapist who works in concert with the IICAPS team.

A second area of intervention in this Domain is related to the assessment and treatment of the behavioral and physical health needs of all other family members, in addition to those of the identified patient. The untreated health and behavioral health problems of family members may negatively affect the Main Problem directly or indirectly. If untreated, such problems may undermine a family member's ability to contribute appropriately to family functioning. Specifically, untreated behavioral health problems may impair a parent's ability to provide leadership, nurturance, and appropriate boundaries and limits. They may also contribute directly to the identified patient's level of symptoms and dyscontrol. In addition, such problems may be a major barrier to the successful implementation of any and all elements of the Treatment Plan. For these reasons, the IICAPS team and family members must carefully evaluate the health and behavioral health needs of all family members while also assessing the impact of these needs on family functioning. After this evaluation is completed, the IICAPS team and family members should develop and implement appropriate Goals and Action Steps to ameliorate the identified health problems.

## SCHOOL DOMAIN

Second only to the family, school provides the major environmental and life experience for children in our culture. Although all children are vulnerable to inadequacies in their school programming, children with SED are more likely to be adversely affected. The IICAPS team, family members, and appropriate school personnel must assess each child's individual educational plan, paying special attention to academic appropriateness, social experiences, and behavioral programming. Following this assessment, the IICAPS team, family members, and school personnel should identify the areas in need of remediation. The remediation plan is then included among the Goals and Action Steps in the School Domain of the Treatment Plan.

## ENVIRONMENT AND OTHER SYSTEMS

The Environment and Other Systems Domain of the Treatment Plan addresses basic life issues such as safety, housing, recreation, and financial condition that create barriers to accessing needed services, produce significant stress for the child and family, and/or exacerbate the Main Problem. For example, grossly inadequate housing creates problems of lack of privacy, poor physical boundaries, health risks, and personal safety. Similarly a lack of access to recreation may stunt social development and increase the stress and irritation of family members, also leading to exacerbation of the Main Problem. The Goals and Action Steps in this Domain are directly linked to ameliorating these deficits.

Addressing the issues in this Domain is a process that might well fit under the rubric of intensive care management. Intensive care management, or case management, has been demonstrated in randomized controlled studies to be associated with significantly improved outcomes as compared to intervention without this service (Farmer, Dorsey, and Mustillo, 2004). In IICAPS the intensive care management is not separated from the other aspects of the intervention. Instead both the planning and implementation are part of the overall Treatment Plan.

## CASE ILLUSTRATION: MARQUIS

### Referral Information

Marquis was a nine-year-old African American male who was referred to IICAPS following a two-week admission to an in-patient child psychiatric unit in a general hospital. Although Marquis had an extensive history of aggression and impulsivity, in the two months before his hospitalization these behaviors had escalated. His admission to the unit followed Marquis's attempt to attack his younger brother with a knife, an event that marked the culmination of his loss of control. At the time of referral to IICAPS, Marquis was living with his adoptive parents, his maternal aunt and uncle, with whom he had lived since three years of age and by whom he was legally adopted at age six. The in-patient unit staff had recommended IICAPS for Marquis and his family because of the severity of his behavioral difficulties and his parents' difficulties in managing his behaviors. Issues of consistent limit setting and excessive physical discipline were singled out for IICAPS attention. In addition, there were serious concerns about Marquis's school placement and the monitoring of his medications.

### Diagnosis

When Marquis began IICAPS treatment he had an Axis I diagnosis of Attention Deficit Hyperactivity Disorder, Combined Type; Oppositional Defiant Disorder; and a rule/out for Bipolar Disorder. His Axis II diagnoses were rule/outs for Specific Learning Disabilities and Borderline Intellectual Functioning. Marquis's Axis III diagnosis was asthma, his Axis IV diagnosis was severe problems with parenting and school, and his Global Assessment of Functioning (GAF) score was 42. His medication upon discharge from the hospital consisted of 36 milligrams of Concerta, a long-acting stimulant administered once a day in the morning.

### The Family

Little is known about Marquis's biologic family or his early history. His mother is thought to have a mental illness, probably Schizophrenia, and is known to be addicted to crack cocaine. It is likely that Marquis was exposed to cocaine *in utero*. At the time of referral to IICAPS it was thought that she had not been in recent contact with Marquis, although this was later found not to be the case. His father's identity and location remain unknown. There is no extant information about Marquis's development prior to his placement with his aunt and uncle, his adoptive parents.

Marquis lived with his adoptive parents, a 6.5-year-old adoptive brother, and a three-year-old adoptive sister. Marquis's adoptive mother presented as overwhelmed and possibly depressed. His father, who worked more than 60 hours per week, was generally unavailable to the family. The household was characterized as stressful, with little meaningful communication between the parents. Yelling or resorting to physicality marked many of the exchanges between parents and children.

## IICAPS Intervention

### ASSESSMENT & ENGAGEMENT PHASE

The initial meeting between the family, the IICAPS team, and the hospital unit staff took place on the in-patient unit two days before Marquis was discharged to home. At that time the IICAPS team established an initial meeting schedule that was to begin immediately following Marquis's return to his family. During that first meeting, one team member met with the parents, the other with the children. In response to questions about what problems they wanted to address with the team immediately, both parents stated that they wanted to meet with the school to plan for an appropriate school placement for Marquis. They also wanted to arrange a meeting with a child psychiatrist for assessment and medication for him. The team appreciated the fact that the family's goals were consistent with those noted by the hospital staff at the time of referral.

The tools used during this phase provided further information about child and family functioning. In the process of identifying strengths and vulnerabilities, the parents and Marquis stated that he was handsome, in good physical health, athletic, had friends in the neighborhood, and had been in the same school since kindergarten They listed his vulnerabilities as being impulsive, aggressive, angry, having intellectual deficits, and doing poorly in school, where he had had multiple suspensions. The family also enumerated his distrust of adults, his poor attention tolerance, and his stealing as other deficiencies. The family identified its own strengths as being intact, committed to Marquis, hard-working, and having a father who was employed. Other strengths included a supportive, extended paternal family, and the fact that Marquis's 6.5-year-old brother appeared to be developmentally on track. The family believed that the mother's possible depression, the father's unavailability because of his long hours of work, the lack of communication between the parents, the parents' difficulties in setting consistent limits and using excessive discipline, the financial stress under which they lived, and the language delays and emotional neediness of Marquis's three-year-old sister were all deficits that contributed to the family's problems.

The process of gathering information begins during the first session of the Assessment & Engagement Phase and continues throughout the intervention.

The most salient aspect of the process is the engagement of the child and family in the work of treatment. In this case, the family was able to identify those areas of both the child's and the family's lives that were the most troubling to them, thus most available for intervention. Shortly after entering the case, the team coordinated an appointment for Marquis with a child psychiatrist to evaluate his medication. During this Phase, in an effort to encourage Marquis to become involved in prosocial sports activities, the team also worked to enroll him in a basketball program at the local Young Men's Christian Association (YMCA). Simultaneously they began to teach him skills to increase his frustration tolerance and help him to address and manage his anger and aggression. In his regular sessions with a team member he played games designed to help him cope with the distress of losing as well as to experience the pleasure of winning. His family encouraged him to find a quiet place to calm down when he became angry.

In the Family Domain, the team utilized the issues identified by the family as vehicles for deepening the therapeutic relationship. This approach led the team to evaluate the extent of his mother's depression, help both parents with behavioral management and limit setting, begin in-home family therapy, obtain an evaluation of the three-year-old sister's language skills, and recommend consideration of marital counseling to improve communication between Marquis's parents.

In the School Domain, the team learned that the school, which had special education facilities available, was willing to review Marquis's educational plan and schedule a Planning and Placement Team meeting (PPT), an essential element in planning for his educational placement. However, the school had not identified his special needs and had overused suspensions as a way of dealing with his troubling behaviors. Marquis's current teacher was unsympathetic to him, and as a result Marquis's mother did not like her. In fact, children with behavioral health problems frequently overwhelmed the staff of this particular school. The team responded to this situation by advocating strongly for educational and cognitive testing and immediate assistance for Marquis in reading and expressive language. Team members also met with his teacher to help her understand his difficulties and to develop a behavioral plan that would be consistent with a plan they were attempting to set in place at his home.

The following Strengths & Vulnerabilities were identified by the family in the Environmental Domain: the home was clean and well kept, the neighborhood was stable, there was adequate food and clothing for family members,

and the family had a car and had no history of involvement with either protective services or the court. However, the family felt stressed financially and
isolated from social supports. The father took the car to work while the mother
and children relied on public transportation to attend appointments, an additional stressor. The team was able to help the father adjust his schedule so that
on days when the mother and children needed to keep appointments he would
find alternative transportation. In addition, the team scheduled a late-evening
meeting each week so that the father could be included in the sessions.

The Assessment & Engagement Phase ended with the creation of the
Treatment Plan that signaled the beginning of the Work & Action Phase. By
this time the family had already experienced some movement toward their
own goals and were ready to engage more fully and more authentically in
the work.

WORK & ACTION PHASE

Throughout this Phase interventions are tried and modified in an iterative
fashion to reflect the acquisition of additional information and the success
or lack of success of particular treatment approaches. By the start of this
Phase the IICAPS team learned that Marquis's biologic mother had reap-
peared in his life six months before his hospitalization. Although she had had
no contact with Marquis for two years preceding her reappearance, she began
placing frequent telephone calls to him that resulted in several conversations
between them. These conversations were difficult for Marquis, and as a result the adoptive parents tried to prevent their occurrence. When Marquis
received a call from his mother during the intervention, the team was able
to observe the full extent of his emotional and behavioral decompensation.
The team hypothesized that Marquis's ambivalence toward his mother played
an important role in his behavior in general and was specifically significant
in the decline that was precipitated by actual contact with her. As a result,
the team helped the parents to establish rules that would block any contact
between Marquis and his mother and protect him from his own ambivalence and guilt. The family's telephone number was changed, and the parents
requested an order of no contact from the court, which was granted in the
child's interest. Most important, Marquis himself entered outpatient treatment, where he could address his complicated feelings toward both his biologic and adoptive parents.

As the family sessions proceeded, the team became aware that the un-
derlying reasons for the hostility between Marquis's father and mother were

related to the father's perception that his wife had forced him to take in and adopt Marquis. The father believed that if they had not adopted Marquis, his wife would be able to work, and the family's finances would be improved. As these and other family issues were brought into the sessions, the therapeutic surface was expanded significantly, and even more authentic work was able to take place.

The Treatment Plan shown in Figure 5.1 at the end of the case illustration captures the Main Problem, the central focus of the Goals that are established by the family and team in the four IICAPS Domains. The plan represents an attempt to improve the fit between Marquis, his parents, and his siblings by meeting the goals and objectives that they have established for themselves.

Each Attainment Scale is completed by the family with the IICAPS team. The family needs to answer the questions "How successful are we at working on a particular Action Step?" and "How successful are we at reaching a particular Goal?" The family and the team use attainment scaling to measure the child and family's progress toward changing the specific behaviors they have identified as contributors to the child's Main Problem. For example, if the child was wetting his bed every night, the Action Step might be to reduce bed wetting to once a week. Once that was attained, the Action Step might be "no wetting for one month." Figure 5.1 shows Goals and Action Steps with Attainment Scales.

*Family Domain.* During this Phase of treatment a number of family-specific interventions were initiated to assist the family members to meet the Goals they had set. The team introduced a behavioral chart and a system of rewards that the parents agreed to follow. They also agreed that they would no longer use physical punishment. The chart addressed only two behaviors: no hitting and the importance of following directions. The team was able to help the family members adopt rules for settling conflicts and for guiding day-to-day activities that led to improved household functioning. The mother was able to enter into treatment for her depression. With the help of the team, she and her husband were able to address some of the issues that had badly strained their relationship. Marquis's father was able to make travel arrangements twice a week so that his mother could schedule appointments for herself and her children for the times when she had a car.

*School Domain.* Testing revealed that Marquis had a low average I.Q. and was in the learning-disabled range in both reading and writing. Although efforts were made to help his teacher understand his learning deficits and make compensatory arrangements for him, these efforts were not successful. However, the school Planning and Placement Team meeting called by his mother resulted in a decision to move Marquis to another school that could offer him both behavioral health and special educational services.

*Environmental Domain.* Marquis's three-year-old sister was evaluated, and although she had a language delay, it was only in the moderate range, a fact that helped to assuage her mother's anxiety. She was enrolled in a preschool enrichment program that she seemed to look forward to attending. With her daughter in school, the mother began to consider the possibility of finding a part-time job. Neither parent was interested in seeking the financial advice that was recommended by the team.

ENDING & WRAP-UP PHASE

The Ending & Wrap-Up Phase begins when the family's primary treatment Goals are met and the child is no longer at risk of hospitalization. At this point the child and family should be able to engage effectively in appropriate traditional outpatient treatment. At the time that Marquis and his family entered the Ending & Wrap-Up Phase they had achieved their aims and felt more confident of their future.

*Child Domain.* As the case moved toward discharge, Marquis was less aggressive and easier to manage both in school and at home. He was engaged in his outpatient treatment. His medications continued to include 36 milligrams of Concerta once daily in the morning, but he was now also taking 0.1 milligram of Clonidine at bedtime to help with his hyperactivity without causing insomnia. Marquis was continuing to be involved in basketball at the YMCA and was also enrolled in an afterschool program.

*Family Domain.* The mother was now on antidepressant medication as prescribed by her internist. Her depression had lifted, and the level of marital discord had decreased. Both parents were able to use the behavioral chart appropriately and no longer felt the need to use corporal punishment. Marquis's three-year-old sister was no longer as needy as she had been and showed more positive affect.

*School Domain.* Marquis's new school markedly altered his educational experience. The school personnel have a realistic appreciation of Marquis and his needs. They recognize the level of support that he needs and are willing and committed to working with him and his parents. In fact, the school has encouraged his parents' involvement in developing and monitoring his educational plan. The school social worker and his outpatient therapist are in regular contact so that their work with him is coordinated.

*Environmental Domain.* The financial stress that burdened the family has not been relieved. The family is resistant to seeking advice in this area, but the mother is planning to look for part-time work. The family is making good use of traditional outpatient resources. The team left the family after a celebration in which they reviewed their accomplishments and reflected on the progress they had made and the process in which they had been engaged. The family was made aware that the team would welcome a call from time to time to hear how they were doing.

## IICAPS Treatment Plan with Attainment Scales

| Child's Name | Date of Birth | Date of Intake | Date of Treatment Plan/Review |
|---|---|---|---|
| Marquis | September 20, 1994 | August 12, 2003 | |

### Main Problem(s):

*Marquis's angry outbursts, fighting, biting, and trouble in school*

How likely is this behavior to result in hospitalization?

Attainment Scale:  1    2    3    4    5    6    7    8    9    10
          (imminent risk)      (moderate risk)      (low risk)

Goals of Treatment: Each goal is a brief statement in terms that indicate a positive resolution of a problem or need, as seen in a demonstrated new behavior. Goals should be determined by the family with the IICAPS team.

Action Steps: Assignments or tasks; means of realizing treatment goals; states how or what treatments the team will utilize to facilitate a specific change in behavior. The role responsibilities of team members should be clearly stated, i.e., who will do what.

Each Attainment Scale is completed by the family with the IICAPS team. The family needs to answer the question, "How successful are we at doing a particular Action Step?" Also, "How successful are we at reaching a particular goal?" On the attainment scale, replace the word "behavior" with a concrete behavior that exemplifies this level of goal attainment e.g. "wets the bed every night"; "wets the bed once a week"; "no wetting for one month."

### I. Child Domain:

Strengths: *good looking, good health, likes sports, has some friends, been in same school since kindergarten*

Vulnerabilities: *out of control, angry, does poorly in school, doesn't trust grown-ups, doesn't like it when things don't go his way, steals, moody*

Figure 5.1. Treatment Plan with Attainment Scales: Marquis

**Child Goal 1:** *Marquis will control his angry and aggressive impulses so that he can stay at home and in school.*

**How successful are we at reaching the goal?**

| Attainment Scale: | 1 | 2 | 3 | 4 | 5 | 6 | 7 | 8 | 9 | 10 |
|---|---|---|---|---|---|---|---|---|---|---|
| | (behavior) | | | | | (behavior) | | | | (behavior) |
| | No action taken | | | | | | | | | completed |

**Action Step 1.1:** *Marquis will see a psychiatrist to find out about his problems and get medications to treat them.*

| Attainment Scale: | 1 | 2 | 3 | 4 | 5 | 6 | 7 | 8 | 9 | 10 |
|---|---|---|---|---|---|---|---|---|---|---|
| | (behavior) | | | | | (behavior) | | | | (behavior) |
| | Not at all | | | | | | | | | completed |

**Action Step 1.2:** *Marquis will try harder to manage his moods.*

| Attainment Scale: | 1 | 2 | 3 | 4 | 5 | 6 | 7 | 8 | 9 | 10 |
|---|---|---|---|---|---|---|---|---|---|---|
| | (behavior) | | | | | (behavior) | | | | (behavior) |
| | Not at all | | | | | | | | | completed |

**Child Goal 2:** *Marquis will try to do better in sports and with friends.*

**How successful are we at reaching the goal?**

| Attainment Scale: | 1 | 2 | 3 | 4 | 5 | 6 | 7 | 8 | 9 | 10 |
|---|---|---|---|---|---|---|---|---|---|---|
| | (behavior) | | | | | (behavior) | | | | (behavior) |
| | No action taken | | | | | | | | | completed |

**Action Step 2.1:** *Marquis will attend the basketball program at the YMCA.*

| Attainment Scale: | 1 | 2 | 3 | 4 | 5 | 6 | 7 | 8 | 9 | 10 |
|---|---|---|---|---|---|---|---|---|---|---|
| | (behavior) | | | | | (behavior) | | | | (behavior) |
| | Not at all | | | | | | | | | completed |

**Action Step 2.2:** *Marquis will take space in his room when he feels angry. He will not hit his brother or sister.*

| Attainment Scale: | 1 | 2 | 3 | 4 | 5 | 6 | 7 | 8 | 9 | 10 |
|---|---|---|---|---|---|---|---|---|---|---|
| | (behavior) | | | | | (behavior) | | | | (behavior) |
| | Not at all | | | | | | | | | completed |

## II. Child and Family Domain:

Strengths: *intact family, they love Marquis and want him to do better, father employed, brother doing well developmentally, father's extended family is supportive*

Vulnerabilities: *Mother is overwhelmed, father is often unavailable because of work hours, little communication between parents, difficulties setting limits or sticking with rules, sister may have language delay*

**Family Goal 1:** *Parents will do better enforcing the limits and rules they set.*

**How successful are we at reaching the goal?**

| Attainment Scale: | 1 | 2 | 3 | 4 | 5 | 6 | 7 | 8 | 9 | 10 |
|---|---|---|---|---|---|---|---|---|---|---|
| | (behavior) | | | | | (behavior) | | | | (behavior) |
| | No action taken | | | | | | | | | completed |

**Action Step 1.1:** *Parents will work with team to create rules, routines and rituals that Marquis and the other children can count on.*

| Attainment Scale: | 1 | 2 | 3 | 4 | 5 | 6 | 7 | 8 | 9 | 10 |
|---|---|---|---|---|---|---|---|---|---|---|
| | (behavior) | | | | | (behavior) | | | | (behavior) |
| | Not at all | | | | | | | | | completed |

**Action Step 1.2:** *Parents will recognize early signs of Marquis's troubling behaviors and learn how to keep things from getting worse.*

| Attainment Scale: | 1 | 2 | 3 | 4 | 5 | 6 | 7 | 8 | 9 | 10 |
|---|---|---|---|---|---|---|---|---|---|---|
| | (behavior) | | | | | (behavior) | | | | (behavior) |
| | Not at all | | | | | | | | | completed |

**Family Goal 2:** *Family members will understand more about each one's needs and try to respond to each other more appropriately.*

**How successful are we at reaching the goal?**

| Attainment Scale: | 1 | 2 | 3 | 4 | 5 | 6 | 7 | 8 | 9 | 10 |
|---|---|---|---|---|---|---|---|---|---|---|
| | (behavior) | | | | | (behavior) | | | | (behavior) |
| | No action taken | | | | | | | | | completed |

**Action Step 2.1:** *Family members will meet together with the team each week and talk about their activities and their feelings.*

| Attainment Scale: | 1 | 2 | 3 | 4 | 5 | 6 | 7 | 8 | 9 | 10 |
|---|---|---|---|---|---|---|---|---|---|---|
| | (behavior) | | | | (behavior) | | | | (behavior) | |
| | Not at all | | | | | | | | completed | |

## III. Child/School Domain:

Strengths: *Marquis has been in the same school since kindergarten. The school is willing to review his educational plan and schedule a PPT. There are special educational facilities at the school.*

Vulnerabilities: *School has not identified Marquis's special needs, school overuses suspension, current teacher is not understanding and Marquis's mother does not like her. Mother feels that school does not work well with children with behavioral health problems.*

**School Goal 1:** *Marquis will be placed in an appropriate school setting.*

**How successful are we at reaching the goal?**

| Attainment Scale: | 1 | 2 | 3 | 4 | 5 | 6 | 7 | 8 | 9 | 10 |
|---|---|---|---|---|---|---|---|---|---|---|
| | (behavior) | | | | (behavior) | | | | (behavior) | |
| | No action taken | | | | | | | | completed | |

**Action Step 1.1:** *Mother should schedule a PPT as soon as possible.*

| Attainment Scale: | 1 | 2 | 3 | 4 | 5 | 6 | 7 | 8 | 9 | 10 |
|---|---|---|---|---|---|---|---|---|---|---|
| | (behavior) | | | | (behavior) | | | | (behavior) | |
| | Not at all | | | | | | | | completed | |

**Action Step 1.2:** *Mother should request educational and cognitive testing and help in reading.*

| Attainment Scale: | 1 | 2 | 3 | 4 | 5 | 6 | 7 | 8 | 9 | 10 |
|---|---|---|---|---|---|---|---|---|---|---|
| | (behavior) | | | | (behavior) | | | | (behavior) | |
| | Not at all | | | | | | | | completed | |

**School Goal 2:** *Improve teacher's understanding of Marquis.*

**How successful are we at reaching the goal?**

| Attainment Scale: | 1 | 2 | 3 | 4 | 5 | 6 | 7 | 8 | 9 | 10 |
|---|---|---|---|---|---|---|---|---|---|---|
| | (behavior) | | | | (behavior) | | | | (behavior) | |
| | No action taken | | | | | | | | completed | |

**Action Step 2.1:** *Mother and team should meet with teacher.*

| Attainment Scale: | 1 | 2 | 3 | 4 | 5 | 6 | 7 | 8 | 9 | 10 |
|---|---|---|---|---|---|---|---|---|---|---|
| | (behavior) | | | | (behavior) | | | | (behavior) | |
| | Not at all | | | | | | | | | completed |

**Action Step 2.2:** *Mother and Team should encourage teacher to use a behavioral plan for Marquis that is similar to the plan that mother will use at home.*

| Attainment Scale: | 1 | 2 | 3 | 4 | 5 | 6 | 7 | 8 | 9 | 10 |
|---|---|---|---|---|---|---|---|---|---|---|
| | (behavior) | | | | (behavior) | | | | (behavior) | |
| | Not at all | | | | | | | | | completed |

## IV. Physical Environment and Other Systems Domain (including adequacy of housing, and extended support systems):

Strengths: *Home is clean and well kept. Neighborhood is stable, not overly dangerous. Family has the food and clothing it needs. Family has one car. Family has never been involved with protective services or the court.*

Vulnerabilities: *Family is financially stressed. Mother is socially isolated except for paternal extended family. Father takes car, mother has to use public transportation.*

**Physical Environment and Other Systems Goal 1:** *Mother and father will work together to reduce stress and disappointment in the family.*

**How successful are we at reaching the goal?**

| Attainment Scale: | 1 | 2 | 3 | 4 | 5 | 6 | 7 | 8 | 9 | 10 |
|---|---|---|---|---|---|---|---|---|---|---|
| | (behavior) | | | | (behavior) | | | | (behavior) | |
| | No action taken | | | | | | | | | completed |

**Action Step 1.1:** *Father and mother will work out use of car.*

| Attainment Scale: | 1 | 2 | 3 | 4 | 5 | 6 | 7 | 8 | 9 | 10 |
|---|---|---|---|---|---|---|---|---|---|---|
| | (behavior) | | | | (behavior) | | | | (behavior) | |
| | Not at all | | | | | | | | | completed |

**Action Step 1.2:** *Parents will work on issues of budgeting and finances.*

| Attainment Scale: | 1 | 2 | 3 | 4 | 5 | 6 | 7 | 8 | 9 | 10 |
|---|---|---|---|---|---|---|---|---|---|---|
| | (behavior) | | | | (behavior) | | | | (behavior) | |
| | Not at all | | | | | | | | | completed |

**Physical Environment and Other Systems Goal 2:** *Mother will take steps to become more involved in activities outside of the home.*

**How successful are we at reaching the goal?**

| Attainment Scale: | 1 | 2 | 3 | 4 | 5 | 6 | 7 | 8 | 9 | 10 |
|---|---|---|---|---|---|---|---|---|---|---|
| | (behavior) | | | | (behavior) | | | | (behavior) | |
| | No action taken | | | | | | | | | completed |

**Action Step 2.1:** *Mother will make an attempt to spend time with others and enroll in a parent support group.*

| Attainment Scale: | 1 | 2 | 3 | 4 | 5 | 6 | 7 | 8 | 9 | 10 |
|---|---|---|---|---|---|---|---|---|---|---|
| | (behavior) | | | | (behavior) | | | | (behavior) | |
| | Not at all | | | | | | | | | completed |

**Action Step 2.2:** *Mother will set up an appointment with a therapist.*

| Attainment Scale: | 1 | 2 | 3 | 4 | 5 | 6 | 7 | 8 | 9 | 10 |
|---|---|---|---|---|---|---|---|---|---|---|
| | (behavior) | | | | (behavior) | | | | (behavior) | |
| | Not at all | | | | | | | | | completed |

## Summary of Goals (group goals by domain):

**Child:** *Marquis will control his angry and destructive behaviors so that he can stay at home and in school. Marquis will work on and improve his ability to make friends with other children and take part in outside activities and sports.*

**Family:** *Parents will improve their parenting and limit setting skills. Family members will understand each other better and change their attitudes and behaviors towards each other.*

**School:** *Marquis will be placed in an appropriate school setting. Mother and Team will attempt to improve teacher's understanding of Marquis.*

**Physical Environment and Other Systems:** *Family stress will be relieved through talking and planning together. Mother will take steps to get involved in activities outside of the house.*

**Signatures:**

Parent :_____    Date: _____

Parent :_____    Date: _____

Child   :_____    Date: _____

Clinician:_____    Date: _____

**Mental Health Counselor :**_____  **Date:** _____
**Supervisor** _____  **Date:** _____

# Chapter 6  Special Clinical Issues

There are some special clinical problems that, when they become known to the IICAPS team, require a sharper focus or an alteration of the Treatment Plan. Although each child and family should be understood in light of their unique strengths and vulnerabilities, the evolving developmental psychopathology and treatment literatures have identified specific issues that benefit from special consideration. These issues must be addressed if treatment is to progress and the Goals of the Treatment Plan are to be attained.

## DOMESTIC VIOLENCE

Violence is not unusual in troubled families. Many individuals and families resort to violence as a basic mode of communication and problem solving and as an attempt to gain control or to satisfy needs. Domestic violence may be especially prevalent in families in which there is significant psychopathology coupled with intellectual disability and serious problems of impulse control. One of the more toxic and insidious forms of violence to which children are subjected is intimate partner violence. The correlation between exposure to domestic violence and childhood psychopathology is indisputable. In families in which domestic violence occurs, the rates of childhood anxiety, mood, and disruptive behavior disorders are greater than the rates for the general population. Research findings also suggest that rates of child abuse are elevated between 30 percent and 60 percent in families that experience domestic violence (Osofsky, 1999).

When a family is affected by domestic violence, the unwanted behavior should become the primary focus of the IICAPS intervention. Intrafamilial violence is never acceptable, and its negative impact on child development and mental health is inarguable. Without a sense of safety and bodily integrity, no child can engage freely in treatment. To promote a sense of safety as quickly as possible, the IICAPS team must work with the parents to ensure that all potential weapons are removed from the household. In addition, safety plans should be developed with the family, and rules for containment should be drafted.

Generally, it is expected that when necessary the perpetrator and not the victim should be removed from the household. However, the child's sense of safety is not assured simply by the fact that the domestic violence perpetrator is no longer living in the home. In some cases family members continue to be in overt or covert contact with the perpetrator and may express anger toward the child or the mother if either acted as the accuser. In other cases one or more family members may behave in ways that mimic the perpetrator's threatening behaviors, thus maintaining the child's anxiety and concern. The complexity of these behaviors, reflecting as they do the relationships and needs of all members of the family, adds to the difficulties inherent in working with families in which children are affected by domestic violence. The elimination of domestic violence is generally a slow, multistep process. The work requires an understanding of and intervention with the multifactorial processes that have sustained the noxious behaviors over time. To increase their effectiveness in helping families to address domestic violence, IICAPS teams are encouraged to include local police authorities, courts, child protective services, and other community programs as collaborators in the intervention.

### Case Illustration: Michael

REFERRAL INFORMATION

Michael was a 12-year-old Caucasian boy referred to IICAPS after his second hospitalization within three months for aggressive and dangerous behavior that was unresponsive to medication trials and psychotherapy. He lived with his mother, Alice, and two younger sisters in a solidly middle-class neighborhood. His father, John, had been out of the house for two years for violence he perpetrated against Michael's mother. Previously incarcerated for six months on charges of domestic violence, when Michael was referred to IICAPS, John was out of jail and living with his own parents.

DIAGNOSIS

At the time of referral Michael had Axis I diagnoses of Oppositional Defiant Disorder and Intermittent Explosive Disorder with a rule/out of Bipolar Disorder. He had no Axis II conditions. He was in good health but was suffering from severe difficulties with his primary support group that were thought to be sequelae of his exposure to domestic violence. He had been given a GAF score of 38. When discharged from the hospital, Michael was taking 500 milligrams of Valproate twice daily for his mood disorder. Michael had entered outpatient psychotherapy when he was nine years old, but stopped after several months. He had restarted treatment one month before his first hospitalization.

Michael was of average intelligence and did not have any apparent learning disabilities, although his grades had been poor from the time he entered school. His school considered him an underachiever, and his teachers often accused him of being lazy and disruptive. Michael had friends in both his school and neighborhood and was at his best when playing sports or riding his bicycle.

THE FAMILY

Michael's mother was both passive and anxious. She was unable to provide appropriate structure, boundaries, or limits for any of her three children. When Michael was hospitalized, Michael's mother visited him frequently and was actively involved in his treatment. However, when he returned home from the hospital his outpatient clinician found that she was unreliable and forgetful. As a result, Michael missed several clinic appointments, and his treatment did not go well.

Relationships among the siblings were conflicted. Michael's sisters did not share his angry feelings about their father. Additionally, the family was involved with the state child protective service agency as a result of multiple reports of domestic violence and an unsubstantiated accusation of child abuse.

## IICAPS Intervention

ASSESSMENT & ENGAGEMENT PHASE

The initial stages of the assessment revealed to the IICAPS team that the family's long history of domestic violence was continuing to influence all aspects of their lives. Michael's mother and her children were fearful that their father would return to the home after his release from jail. Michael's mother, who met criteria for Post-Traumatic Stress Disorder (PTSD), had become increasingly withdrawn and depressed since his release. She had been unable to maintain her job, her unemployment benefits were due to expire, she was unable to pay her bills, and she was worried that she would lose her house, which technically she still co-owned with her husband. Although Michael's mother wanted to pursue a divorce, she had not initiated any action for fear that her husband would become enraged and attack her physically.

Michael's mother identified Michael with his father. She told the team that although Michael had always been a difficult child to manage he had become even more difficult during the past year. She described Michael as moody and sullen. He would often hit his mother when his wishes were thwarted, although these actions would be followed by remorse. Michael's aggression was directed only toward his mother, not toward his sisters or his friends. Michael left his house at every opportunity, going outside to play or to the home of a friend. He would stay away as long as possible, often disregarding the time he was told to return.

Michael himself presented as a very worried, angry, and sad boy. He told the IICAPS team that he hated his father and disliked his mother even more. In family sessions he would sit silently or demand to go outside with one of the IICAPS team members to play basketball. The IICAPS team believed that Michael was worried that his father might return to the family and that his mother would not be able to stop him. His mother's inability to protect herself or her children from their father's anger and physical abuse infuriated Michael. His increased aggression was the product of his frustration and fear.

Michael's sisters had very different feelings about their father, whom they idealized. His sisters stated explicitly that they would rather live with their father than with their mother. They had never directly witnessed any episodes of domestic violence, although they were aware that it had taken place. The details of their mother's injuries were unknown to them. They perceived their mother as incompetent and ineffectual and fantasized that their father would be more reliable and available to them.

As the Assessment & Engagement Phase continued, important information emerged. The IICAPS team learned that since his release from jail, Michael's father had been making threatening telephone calls to Michael's mother regularly. Even though she had an unlisted telephone and had changed her number several times, Michael's father managed to obtain the new number and continued to harass her. Although Michael's mother told the team that she found evidence that her husband had actually come into the house on at least two occasions, she did not tell the children that this had occurred.

The IICAPS team worked closely with Michael's mother to allow the range of feelings that family members had about Michael's father to become more transparent. However, his mother was reluctant to discuss her history of domestic violence and harassment with her children for fear that they would become "upset." While she did not really want them to have an ongoing relationship with their father, she also stated that she didn't want her feelings about him to "contaminate" those of her children. When the IICAPS team brought up the possibility of contacting the authorities about the harassing phone calls and the break-ins, she adamantly refused and would not allow any further discussion. During this time, Michael's behavior at home continued to be aggressive and oppositional, and his mother continued to be withdrawn and isolative.

### WORK & ACTION PHASE

The initial Phase of intervention culminated in the family's realization that despite the father's absence from the home and the elimination of violence between Michael's parents, the specter of the father, the potential for future violence, and the treatment of mother's post-traumatic symptoms were the key to Michael's treatment. In the IICAPS model, the end of the Assessment & Engagement Phase is marked by the creation of a Treatment Plan, which then guides the work of the second Phase of IICAPS intervention, Work & Action. Michael and his family were now ready to develop such a plan.

The Treatment Plan is a document designed to significantly reduce the likelihood that the Main Problem, in this case Michael's aggressive and potentially dangerous behaviors, will place him at risk of further hospitalization. In the process of developing the Treatment Plan and identifying the Goals the family wished to attain with the help of the IICAPS team, Michael and his mother recognized that no real progress could occur until Michael was able to feel safe and secure at home. With this fact in mind, the team together with Michael and his mother created a short, focused Treatment Plan that the team hoped would lead eventually to more therapeutically oriented Goals & Action Steps as the intervention progressed.

The IICAPS team believed that keeping Michael occupied outside his home would reduce his contact with his mother, help to contain his aggression, and decrease the stress they each experienced. The team hypothesized that Michael's anxiety, which was expressed in his fights with his mother, often mirrored her own anxious feelings. Family therapy, a usual IICAPS intervention, was not possible at this point because of the instability of the family. Instead, the lead clinician was to work with Michael's mother individually to help her address her own feelings and worries and understand her possible role in creation of a more stable home environment. The Treatment Plan shown in Figure 6.1 at the end of the case illustration describes the Goals set by the family in the four Domains addressed by IICAPS. The plan represents an attempt to help Michael's mother to play an executive, more empowered role in Michael's life at home and at school. The plan was designed to reduce Michael's anxiety at home and to enlist more support for him at school. The ultimate goal was to reduce his aggression and lack of impulse control so that he would no longer engage in potentially dangerous behaviors. Other important family stressors such as their troubled financial status were also addressed.

*Child Domain.* Michael was eager to work on plans for activities outside his home. He expressed an interest in several sports activities and decided to pursue basketball. The team was able to obtain a scholarship for Michael at the local YMCA and encouraged him to enroll in the basketball program there. Michael refused to participate in the program; he believed that the YMCA was a terrible place and only losers went there. Unfortunately, there were no other affordable sports options in his community. However, when the IICAPS team discovered that a new basketball league was starting at the YMCA, they contacted one of the coaches and requested that he recruit Michael for the team most appropriate for his age group. The coach was responsive to Michael's situation and followed through on the request. Michael did not refuse the invitation. Somewhat reluctantly he joined the new team. As Michael became actively involved in the basketball league, he became increasingly interested in some of the other activities and programs at the YMCA that he had previously resisted. As expected by the team, his involvement in more prosocial activities outside his home helped to alleviate some of the tension between him and his mother, and there were fewer violent episodes between them.

*Family Domain.* Michael's mother was not ready to engage in psychotherapy with the IICAPS team. She was unable to discuss any symptoms other than her fear of her husband and her worry about her precarious financial position.

She even found it hard to discuss her concerns about her children. Early in this Phase of treatment, the lead clinician, in consultation with her supervisor, decided to broach the subject of antidepressant medication. The IICAPS psychiatrist agreed to see her together with the lead clinician and provide a follow-up consultation to her internist. Michael's mother was placed on a selective serotonin reuptake inhibitor for her depression and PTSD symptomology. Over the next several months, Michael's mother demonstrated moderate improvement in mood and some increased energy. Gradually she became less isolative and withdrawn. Concurrently, her work with the IICAPS Team focused on concrete issues such as finding a job, creating a financial plan, and accessing supportive, preventive services from the Department of Social Services. Ultimately Michael's mother was able to obtain financial assistance to help with her utility and mortgage payments. Importantly, she found a cashier's position, which paid little but was something that she could manage.

As the Work & Action Phase progressed, it became possible for the IICAPS team to schedule family meetings in addition to the individual therapy sessions between the lead clinician and Michael's mother. During these family sessions the team helped Michael's mother to gently tell her children about her experiences with their father, even including the recent, harassing phone calls. The team reinforced the idea that safety was the most essential issue for everyone in the family and that each family member could play a role in helping others to feel safe.

During one of the family sessions, Michael's ten-year-old sister disclosed that she had been in contact with their father. She had been giving him their telephone number because she wanted to talk with him. At this point, both daughters admitted talking to their father. Over the next month the team worked with the family to help them express and accept the complicated feelings raised by these admissions. As a result of the work accomplished in the family sessions, Michael's mother granted permission to the team to meet with the children's father and allowed the two girls to begin supervised visitations with him under the auspices of child protective services. The team also helped Michael's mother to tell her children that if she continued to receive harassing phonecalls she would immediately call the police. This information was also communicated to Michael's father. To everyone's surprise the harassing phone calls soon ended. It appeared that the calls were motivated by Michael's father's anger at Michael's mother for keeping him away from his children. Although Michael was also invited to visit with his father he refused to do so.

*School Domain.* The lead clinician worked with the school to understand Michael's difficulties and to create a behavioral plan consistent with his presentation and concerns. When Michael's teachers made an effort to discuss his feelings with him after a particularly disruptive episode, it appeared to have a calming effect. Although such episodes continued to occur in the school setting, they became shorter in duration, and Michael was able to return to the classroom more quickly. However, his academic performance remained below his capacity.

*Environment and Other Systems Domain.* Although the family's financial situation improved, it continued to be precarious. Michael's mother discussed with the team the possibility of selling the house. However, Michael's parents owned the property jointly, and his mother was still unwilling to pursue divorce proceedings and seek a settlement.

ENDING & WRAP-UP PHASE

When the primary goals of the Work & Action Phase were accomplished, the team worked with the family to develop a Discharge Plan. The Ending & Wrap-Up Phase signifies that the child and family no longer need intensive intervention to maintain the child safely at home. Together the family and the team identify those things that should be addressed before the work is completed. Michael, his mother, and his sisters recognized that continued mental health treatment would help to maintain and extend the gains they had made during the IICAPS intervention. Michael and his mother agreed to meet together with a therapist at a community outpatient mental health agency if the IICAPS team would be present. Support for the transition from home-based services to traditional outpatient care constituted the majority of the work that occurred in this phase as both Michael and his mother gained confidence in themselves and learned to cope with the circumstances of their lives more appropriately.

## CHILD ABUSE AND NEGLECT

Child abuse and neglect are similar in many ways to domestic violence. Addressing child abuse and neglect must be a primary goal of IICAPS, since treatment cannot occur in the presence of active abuse and severe neglect. Child abuse and neglect are frequently multigenerational and multifactorial conditions that can be life-threatening or life-damaging. In some cases these

## IICAPS Treatment Plan with Attainment Scales

| Child's Name | Date of Birth | Date of Intake | Date of Treatment Plan/Review |
|---|---|---|---|
| Michael | April 14, 1993 | May 23, 2005 | |

### Main Problem(s):

*Aggressive and dangerous behavior primarily at home*

**How likely is this behavior to result in hospitalization?**

| Attainment Scale: | 1 | 2 | 3 | 4 | 5 | 6 | 7 | 8 | 9 | 10 |
|---|---|---|---|---|---|---|---|---|---|---|
| | (imminent risk) | | | | (moderate risk) | | | | (low risk) | |

Goals of Treatment: Each goal is a brief statement in terms that indicate a positive resolution of a problem or need, as seen in a demonstrated new behavior. Goals should be determined by the family with the IICAPS team.

Action Steps: Assignments or tasks; means of realizing treatment goals; states how or what treatments the team will utilize to facilitate a specific change in behavior. The role responsibilities of team members should be clearly stated i.e. who will do what.

Each Attainment Scale is completed by the family with the IICAPS team. The family needs to answer the question, "How successful are we at doing a particular Action Step?" Also, "How successful are we at reaching a particular goal?" On the attainment scale, replace the word "behavior" with a concrete behavior that exemplifies this level of goal attainment e.g. "wets the bed every night"; "wets the bed once a week"; "no wetting for one month."

### I. Child Domain:

Strengths: *Good athlete, has many friends*

Vulnerabilities: *Moody and angry, does not listen to mother or teachers, does not use language to discuss issues, does not get along well with mother, medications are not helpful, dislikes school and works below his ability*

Figure 6.1. Treatment Plan with Attainment Scales: Michael

**Child Goal 1:** *Michael will identify activities that he enjoys and will participate in organized programs after school and weekends.*

**How successful are we at reaching the goal?**

| Attainment Scale: | 1 | 2 | 3 | 4 | 5 | 6 | 7 | 8 | 9 | 10 |
|---|---|---|---|---|---|---|---|---|---|---|
| | (behavior) | | | | (behavior) | | | | (behavior) | |
| | No action taken | | | | | | | | completed | |

**Action Step 1.1:** *Michael will review activity options with Mr. Jackson and choose 2-3 to become involved with.*

| Attainment Scale: | 1 | 2 | 3 | 4 | 5 | 6 | 7 | 8 | 9 | 10 |
|---|---|---|---|---|---|---|---|---|---|---|
| | (behavior) | | | | (behavior) | | | | (behavior) | |
| | Not at all | | | | | | | | completed | |

**Action Step 1.2:** *Michael will enroll in 2-3 chosen activities.*

| Attainment Scale: | 1 | 2 | 3 | 4 | 5 | 6 | 7 | 8 | 9 | 10 |
|---|---|---|---|---|---|---|---|---|---|---|
| | (behavior) | | | | (behavior) | | | | (behavior) | |
| | Not at all | | | | | | | | completed | |

## II. Child and Family Domain:

Strengths: *Michael's mother is devoted to all three of her children and wants to be a good parent to them. She tries as hard as she can to protect her children.*

Vulnerabilities: *Michael's mother is frequently stressed and overwhelmed. It is often hard to care for her children the way she would like to. Because of this, she is unable to work.*

**Family Goal 1:** *Michael's mother will be better able to meet the needs of her children and her household.*

**How successful are we at reaching the goal?**

| Attainment Scale: | 1 | 2 | 3 | 4 | 5 | 6 | 7 | 8 | 9 | 10 |
|---|---|---|---|---|---|---|---|---|---|---|
| | (behavior) | | | | (behavior) | | | | (behavior) | |
| | No action taken | | | | | | | | completed | |

**Action Step 1.1:** *Michael's mother and Ms. Williams will meet weekly to identify and practice ways that she can feel less stressed and overwhelmed.*

| Attainment Scale: | 1 | 2 | 3 | 4 | 5 | 6 | 7 | 8 | 9 | 10 |
|---|---|---|---|---|---|---|---|---|---|---|
| | (behavior) | | | | (behavior) | | | | | (behavior) |
| | Not at all | | | | | | | | | completed |

**Action Step 1.2:** *Michael's mother and IICAPS team will create a schedule and structure of activities and responsibilities for family members.*

| Attainment Scale: | 1 | 2 | 3 | 4 | 5 | 6 | 7 | 8 | 9 | 10 |
|---|---|---|---|---|---|---|---|---|---|---|
| | (behavior) | | | | (behavior) | | | | | (behavior) |
| | Not at all | | | | | | | | | completed |

## III. Child/School Domain:

Strengths: *Michael goes to school regularly and passes all his classes.*

Vulnerabilities: *Michael gets into trouble in class and does not do as well as he could academically. Teachers say Michael is lazy.*

**School Goal 1:** *Assist school personnel to develop a better understanding of Michael's emotional needs and his underachievement.*

### How successful are we at reaching the goal?

| Attainment Scale: | 1 | 2 | 3 | 4 | 5 | 6 | 7 | 8 | 9 | 10 |
|---|---|---|---|---|---|---|---|---|---|---|
| | (behavior) | | | | (behavior) | | | | | (behavior) |
| | No action taken | | | | | | | | | completed |

**Action Step 1.1:** *Ms. Williams will observe Michael in school and meet with his teacher and guidance counselor following her observation.*

| Attainment Scale: | 1 | 2 | 3 | 4 | 5 | 6 | 7 | 8 | 9 | 10 |
|---|---|---|---|---|---|---|---|---|---|---|
| | (behavior) | | | | (behavior) | | | | | (behavior) |
| | Not at all | | | | | | | | | completed |

**Action Step 1.2:** *Ms. Williams will meet with the school personnel to create a behavioral plan for Michael.*

| Attainment Scale: | 1 | 2 | 3 | 4 | 5 | 6 | 7 | 8 | 9 | 10 |
|---|---|---|---|---|---|---|---|---|---|---|
| | (behavior) | | | | (behavior) | | | | | (behavior) |
| | Not at all | | | | | | | | | completed |

## IV. Physical Environment and Other Systems Domain (including adequacy of housing, and extended support systems):

Strengths: *Family lives in safe neighborhood and people in neighborhood are friendly.*

Vulnerabilities: *Mother has lost job and is financially strapped.*

**Physical Environment and Other Systems Goal 1:** *Team and mother will engage in financial planning in an attempt to reduce financial stress.*

### How successful are we at reaching the goal?

| Attainment Scale: | 1 | 2 | 3 | 4 | 5 | 6 | 7 | 8 | 9 | 10 |
|---|---|---|---|---|---|---|---|---|---|---|
| | (behavior) | | | | (behavior) | | | | (behavior) | |
| | No action taken | | | | | | | | completed | |

**Action Step1.1:** *Mother will find a part-time job that is not stressful.*

| Attainment Scale: | 1 | 2 | 3 | 4 | 5 | 6 | 7 | 8 | 9 | 10 |
|---|---|---|---|---|---|---|---|---|---|---|
| | (behavior) | | | | (behavior) | | | | (behavior) | |
| | Not at all | | | | | | | | completed | |

**Action Step1.2:** *Team will support mother to go to DSS and learn options for support regarding housing and utilities.*

| Attainment Scale: | 1 | 2 | 3 | 4 | 5 | 6 | 7 | 8 | 9 | 10 |
|---|---|---|---|---|---|---|---|---|---|---|
| | (behavior) | | | | (behavior) | | | | (behavior) | |
| | Not at all | | | | | | | | completed | |

## Summary of Goals (group goals by domain):

**Child:** *Michael will identify activities that he enjoys and will participate in organized programs after school and weekends.*

**Family:** *Michael's mother will be better able to meet the needs of her children and her household.*

**School:** *Assist school personnel to develop a better understanding of Michael's emotional needs and his underachievement.*

**Physical Environment and Other Systems:** *Team and mother will engage in financial planning in an attempt to reduce financial stress.*

**Signatures:**

**Parent :**_____  Date: _____
**Parent :**_____  Date: _____
**Child  :**_____  Date: _____
**Clinician:**_____  Date: _____
**Mental Health Counselor :**_____  Date: _____
**Supervisor** _____  Date: _____

conditions may pose a severe threat to the child's sense of safety. Multiple parental risk factors associated with child abuse and neglect include mental illness, substance abuse, physical illness, unemployment, racism, and poverty.

It is likely that many children served by IICAPS will present with emotional and behavioral issues that are causally related to earlier physical abuse or chronic, pervasive neglect. Many families may have been involved in past protective service investigations, received services from child protective services (CPS) workers, or may be under current CPS supervision. Since IICAPS team members are mandated reporters of child abuse and neglect, an active working relationship between the team and the state agency responsible for child protection is essential. In virtually all situations in which the IICAPS team elects to file a child abuse and neglect report, the adult caregiver must be informed before the child protection agency is notified. Usually the IICAPS team member files the abuse report within the presence of the parent to enhance the transparency of the intervention. Only in extreme cases, when the child's immediate well-being or a person's physical safety is endangered should the protective service agency be notified first. In all other cases the IICAPS team and the CPS worker work together to manage risk in the interest of maintaining the child's attachment to his primary caregiver and preventing his placement outside the home.

If the situation requires the arrest or removal of the perpetrator, a number of unintended consequences should be anticipated. As always, the child's best interest is paramount, and the least detrimental alternative needs to be sought. In every case, the IICAPS team must assess the situation that has led to the abuse, consider whether or not it is remediable, and decide if safety concerns dictate removal. If the family cannot maintain the child safely, can an appropriate caregiver be identified from among the child's extended family and social network? Children who experience life-threatening injuries should be removed from their families and placed with adults able to commit to their long-term care.

## DISRUPTIONS OF PERMANENCE

Significant disruptions in the child's sense of permanence, usually resulting from multiple out-of-home placements, often occur within a context of domestic violence and/or child abuse. Both the IICAPS team and the child's adult caregivers must understand that children who have experienced significant disruptions of attachment may exhibit severe maladaptive behaviors that impede the development of a treatment alliance and challenge any and all attempts to build intimate relationships. Any disruption of a child's sense of permanence is so noxious that the affected child is often constantly vigilant for any hint of disruption. Such "hints" may range from discussion of a household move to the possibility of communication with the abuser. As in contexts of domestic violence, child abuse, and parental substance abuse, addressing the child's disrupted sense of permanence must be a top-priority goal of the intervention, since effective treatment with the child cannot occur when this issue is active and the child is unsure about where and with whom he will live.

Some caregivers join together in malignant custody conflicts that can be defined as intense, relentlessly acrimonious relationships related to battles over custody of a child. Although it is common for this situation to occur in the context of a divorce, it can occur in other contexts as well. Such conflicts are extremely deleterious to the child's well-being and preclude engagement and implementation of treatment. In addition to accentuating the child's existing sense of loss related to the break-up of the original family, this conflict confronts the child with the experience that the caregivers are focused on the conflict rather than on his well-being. As with many of the other special clinical issues, no treatment can occur until this malignant custody conflict is resolved.

## CHILDREN WITH CHRONICALLY
## MENTALLY ILL PARENTS

Rutter and others have described children with parents who suffer from chronic mental illness as at elevated risk for psychiatric disorders of their own (Quinton and Rutter, 1984). The genetic, psychological, and environmental factors associated with adult mental illness all contribute to the child's potential vulnerability. Children whose parents have been diagnosed with Schizophrenia, Bipolar Disorder, and some anxiety disorders are themselves at risk of inheriting these disorders. Families headed by a parent with a chronic mental illness are more likely than other families to live in poor socioeconomic situations. Children in these families are less likely to be monitored and supervised adequately and so may be exposed to more adverse life events. In many affected families older children may assume more of the caretaking role, especially if the ill parent is the mother. In some such families, the parentified child cares not only for the younger children but also for the ill mother (ibid.). On occasion, a pathological enmeshment occurs between the caretaking child and the parent that blurs the boundaries between mother and child and becomes a barrier to appropriate separation and identity formation. In two-parent families with an ill parent, the healthier partner may attempt to compensate for the other's deficits in a maladaptive manner that further derails the child's development.

IICAPS treatment may be complicated by the presence of severe psychopathology in family members other than the identified patient. In these situations, a psychiatric evaluation and treatment with appropriate psychotropic medications and psychotherapies should be supported. IICAPS teams are able to provide individual as well as family therapy to all family members during the course of the intervention. It is expected that if family members are already working with community-based mental health providers they will continue to do so. In addition, IICAPS teams may refer families to other resources that are able to serve the family beyond the period of IICAPS intervention. While siblings may have psychiatric symptoms and difficulties that require immediate attention, parental issues are of particular concern, as parental functioning impacts significantly all members of the family. While the possible manifestations of severe psychopathology may take many forms, there are several that are common and disruptive enough to be addressed here.

Imminent risk of suicide is a life-threatening crisis that takes precedence over other clinical concerns, regardless of which family member is suicidal. When there is a concern about possible suicide, team members must make a careful assessment of suicide risk factors, paying particular attention to the presence of a lethal plan and a means to carry out that plan. If a suicide attempt appears likely, the team and other family members must make and implement a prevention plan. As in any other potentially dangerous situation, safety is the primary concern. If there is any doubt about the individual's safety, he or she should be taken to the hospital emergency department and evaluated (this evaluation may be performed by the IICAPS psychiatrist, if available). However, whenever possible, it is preferable for the IICAPS clinician to perform an assessment in the home before or in lieu of the individual's being taken to a hospital for assessment.

Chronic psychotic illness may affect the identified child, siblings, parents, or other family members simultaneously. Little effective treatment can occur with the affected individual as long as the psychosis is active. If the affected individual is the identified child and/or the parents, then the first focus of treatment must be ameliorating the psychotic process. The current state-of-the-art treatment of psychosis includes antipsychotic medication, stress reduction, and an increase in psychosocial structure. Presumably if the identified child is the only family member who is psychotic, the adult caregivers will be highly motivated to develop an appropriate treatment plan for the psychosis. If one or both of the parents are psychotic, then engaging them in such a treatment plan is generally challenging. However, such engagement is essential if any further treatment is to be possible. When a parent is deemed to be floridly psychotic and unable to function, the team in collaboration with other family members must facilitate a psychiatric hospitalization. Any plan for hospitalization must include an appropriate caretaking arrangement for the child and his siblings.

Working with parents with Paranoia requires a great deal of patience and trust building before any treatment alliance can be achieved and a referral for appropriate psychiatric treatment can be accepted. In some cases a spouse or another family member can assist in this process. However, the nature of the paranoid process may prevent the parent from accessing psychiatric services. In such cases, IICAPS intervention may fail, and it may become necessary to consider a referral to child protective services.

Parental Depression may have as profound an effect on child and family functioning as parental Psychosis. When the team identifies severe parental depressive illness it is necessary for team members to refer the parent for treatment as soon as possible. Additionally, the team should assess the risk of suicidality and determine if hospitalization is appropriate. As with parental Psychosis, any plan for hospitalization should include planning for caretaking of all dependent members of the family.

Parents and caregivers with Mental Retardation and Pervasive Developmental Disorders can create significant barriers to both engagement with the IICAPS team and implementation of the treatment plan. Every aspect of the IICAPS intervention with families presenting with these disorders should be informed by knowledge of the consequences of cognitive and social impairment. The pace of the intervention may need to be slowed, and specific elements of the treatment plan may need to be simplified. As with chronic psychotic illness, the impact of mental retardation and developmental disorders is greatest when one or both parents are affected, since engagement and implementation of the treatment plan may well be compromised.

Active engagement in addictive behavior, including but not limited to drug or alcohol abuse/dependence by important family members, precludes both authentic engagement with the IICAPS team and the work of treatment. Addictive behaviors are especially problematic under the following circumstances: when the engagement in addictive behavior has a higher priority than any other activity, including implementation of the treatment plan; when transparency and truthfulness are sacrificed because of the covert behavior associated with addiction; and when the basic integrity and continuity of the household may have been compromised by illegal behaviors.

The presumption for the IICAPS team should be that no authentic treatment will occur as long as important family members are engaged in addictive behaviors. Thus the first step is to have all relevant family members acknowledge the addictive behavior and move toward the implementation of a plan to address this behavior.

### Case Illustration: Alex

REFERRAL INFORMATION

When referred to IICAPS, Alex, an eight-year-old Caucasian boy, had been hospitalized after attempting to jump out of his third-story apartment window. He reported hearing a voice telling him to jump. During the hospitalization, Alex was found to have frequent auditory hallucinations, a thought disorder, and Borderline Intellectual Functioning. He had frequent aggressive outbursts, panic attacks, and episodes of inconsolable crying. Antipsychotic medication only partially improved these symptoms. However, those that remained were infrequent and less severe. Exposure to stressful situations was found to exacerbate his symptoms.

Alex had not done well in school for some time. He had recently been transferred to a special public school for children in need of behavioral management but was doing poorly there as well. He was restrained at school after a serious aggressive outburst on the same day he attempted to jump out the window.

DIAGNOSIS

At the time of discharge from the hospital and referral to IICAPS Alex had an Axis I diagnosis of Psychotic Disorder, Not Otherwise Specified (NOS), with a rule/out of Schizophrenia, Undifferentiated Type. His Axis II diagnosis was Borderline Intellectual Functioning. He suffered from mild asthma; his environmental stressors were mild. He was given a GAF score of 32. Alex's medications at discharge were 1 milligram of Risperidone in the morning and at noon, and another 2 milligrams at night.

THE FAMILY

Alex's family consisted of his mother, father, two older sisters, ages 14 and 12, and himself. Alex's mother reported that she was overwhelmed by her responsibilities, which included taking care of the family, especially her husband and Alex, and working full-time as a hospital nurse. Alex's father had been diagnosed with Schizophrenia, Paranoid Type, when Alex was two years old. His mother was reported to be anxious and depressed. During the time Alex was hospitalized, he was visited by his mother and occasionally by his sisters, who attended one family session on the in-patient unit. Alex's father never visited his son.

The reasons given by the hospital staff for Alex's referral to IICAPS were to improve the ability of his parents, especially his mother, to parent him effectively and to reduce the level of stress in the home. There were concerns about his mother's feelings of being overwhelmed and her possible overuse of corporal punishment. In addition, the in-patient staff had concerns about the appropriateness of Alex's school placement.

## IICAPS Intervention

ASSESSMENT & ENGAGEMENT PHASE

On their initial visit to the family's residence, the IICAPS team was struck by how clean and orderly the apartment appeared. Although the team found the behavior of Alex's father to be engaging and appropriate during this and subsequent visits in this phase of treatment, he was frequently interrupted by his wife and prevented from voicing his own opinion. Alex's mother appeared to dominate and control all aspects of the family's life and seemed unable or unwilling to share any of her responsibilities. By her own report, Alex's mother slept only four hours each night because she had so much to do. She alone made every meal, did the laundry, and cleaned the house. She expected her children to adhere to her standards in keeping their rooms neat and clean.

Alex's father, who had been a manager in a department store before his psychotic break, was unable to work. His Social Security benefits were his only source of income. Although it became evident to the team that he was more impaired than they initially believed, if permitted by Alex's mother he was capable of providing far more help in managing the children and the household. At the time his activities included watching television, taking out the garbage, and washing the dishes. Although he was at home throughout the day, he had no other responsibilities.

During this phase, Alex's behavior and symptoms fluctuated. Episodes of volatility in school would be followed by problem behaviors upon his return home. During a family session in which the family described a typical 24-hour day, the team learned that Alex was essentially cared for after school by one of his sisters, who would prepare a snack for him and review his homework. For the remainder of the afternoon until his mother returned from work, Alex and his father watched cartoons together. During family sessions, Alex's sisters identified with their mother and joined with her to prevent their father from active participation. They consistently attempted to marginalize their father's role in the family and to minimize the amount of time that he spent together with Alex.

The creation of an intergenerational Genogram, one of the Tools used to guide the Assessment & Engagement Phase, revealed the extensive psychiatric histories on both sides of Alex's family. A number of Alex's paternal relatives carried diagnoses of Psychosis NOS and Bipolar Disorder. Among his maternal relatives there were a significant number of family members with Depressive and Anxiety Disorders. In the process of reconstructing the family's history, Alex's mother revealed her own treatment for depression as an adolescent, which had been unknown to the family until then. The IICAPS team began to understand that her controlling behavior was her way of coping with periods of increased environmental stress and of managing the attendant anxiety and depression that threatened to overwhelm her. By becoming overactive and taking charge of the household, Alex's mother was able to gain some control of her anxiety. She was unaware that her behavior served to increase her own stress, which in turn exacerbated Alex's aggressive actions. The team believed that Alex's mother's anxiety about her husband's psychiatric illness reduced her willingness to involve him in the care of Alex and his sisters. As a result, although Alex wanted his father's support, he was afraid of seeking it out and offending his stressed and demanding mother. Alex's sisters, who were closely allied with their mother, also contributed to the infantilization of both Alex and his father.

WORK & ACTION PHASE

The team and the family entered the Work & Action Phase realizing that each member of the family had a role in doing the work that was expected to reduce Alex's aggressive and out-of-control behaviors and lessen his risk for psychiatric hospitalization. The Treatment Plan shown in Figure 6.2 at the end of the case illustration contains the Goals set by the family with the team in the four IICAPS Domains. Because there was consensus among all family members that Alex would benefit from a change in his school placement, work in the School Domain provided an opportunity to simultaneously engage Alex's mother and increase the involvement of his father in his care. In addition, both parents agreed to work together on techniques that could be used to manage Alex's behavior.

*School Domain.* Because Alex was currently in treatment with a therapist in the community and was also being seen by a community child psychiatrist, the IICAPS team began the Work & Action Phase focusing on those areas essential to Alex's recovery that were not being addressed elsewhere. As a result, the initial work of this Phase focused on finding an appropriate school placement for him. The team's approach was to engage Alex's mother in this process and support her to become an advocate for his educational needs. The team believed that by focusing initially on a concrete task it would be easier for Alex's mother to become comfortable with the team and gain sufficient trust to eventually deal with some of the psychological issues that affected her behavior.

*Family Domain.* The team found that with Alex's mother's attention and energy directed toward his school placement, they were able to restructure the roles played by other family members. The aim of family restructuring was to provide an improved support network for Alex. To that end, the team hoped that Alex's father could play a more direct and supportive role in his care. The team worked on the development of parenting skills with Alex's father individually and also met regularly with both parents on behavioral management technique.

The lead clinician's work with Alex's mother went well. Alex's mother was successful in advocating for his enrollment in a therapeutic school, and she was also able to expand the therapeutic surface to include her own anxiety and depression. As the team had hoped, she agreed to enter into her own treatment. This process occurred over a period of several months during which Alex's mother appeared less stressed and more relaxed. However, the team also recognized that Alex's father would not be able to function appropriately in a parenting role. Unfortunately, he was not able to cope with the stress that resulted from his interactions with Alex and led to his further disorganization and eventual withdrawal from his son. As the limitations of Alex's father became evident, the plan was revised to help him become a more effective and efficient housekeeper. Alex's father began to cook the family's meals, and with some assistance from his family he cleaned the house as well. While neither his cooking nor cleaning was up to his wife's high standards, Alex's mother was now able to assist rather than replace him in these activities. With the restructuring of the family system, Alex's behavior at home began to improve. The change in his school and his enrollment in an extended day program affiliated with the school resulted in even more significant behavioral changes. In addition, much to the delight of her daughters, their mother subsequently gave them permission to participate in extracurricular activities.

ENDING & WRAP-UP PHASE

When the Goals that were established as part of the Treatment Plan were met, the team introduced the idea of ending the Work & Action Phase and moving to the Ending & Wrap-Up Phase. The only logistical issues remaining to be addressed appeared to be related to Alex's mental health treatment and schooling. However, as the team and family approached their final session Alex's father became floridly psychotic and required hospitalization. Almost immediately Alex's behavior deteriorated, and he reported having more hallucinations. In response, the IICAPS team postponed the planned ending. Instead the team helped the family to treat this event as a crisis, but one that they could overcome.

While Alex's father was hospitalized the team learned that he had stopped taking his medication but was initially unable to provide an explanation for his action. Only when the IICAPS team visited him in the hospital did he state that he had stopped taking his medication because he didn't want the team to leave. Upon further exploration of his behavior with the team, Alex's father revealed that he was worried that if the team left the family everything would go back to the way it had been before they came into the family's life. The next day the team met with both of Alex's parents. Alex's mother assured her husband that she wanted things to remain as they were. She was happy that he was able to contribute so much to the running of the household. A few days later, Alex's father returned home. Shortly thereafter, Alex's symptoms and behavior improved. It is likely that an increase in his Risperidone dose also contributed to his improvement. In a subsequent family meeting, Alex disclosed that because everyone appeared so upset at the time of his father's hospitalization, he worried that his father had left the family and would not be returning. The team realized that no one had helped Alex understand what was happening around him. Although he had been told that his father needed to go to the hospital, he hadn't been invited to visit him there. In fact, he did not know where his father was. The crisis provided an opportunity for the family to learn the importance of giving Alex the information and understanding he needed to cope with his anxiety. When this work was accomplished, the team was able to leave Alex and his family.

## ADOLESCENTS IN THE JUVENILE JUSTICE SYSTEM

Adolescents who enter the juvenile justice system may have exhibited problems of affect regulation, impulsivity, and aggression earlier in their development. Better tolerated during childhood, these behaviors are not accepted by their families and communities as youths grow older and become more difficult to manage. Fighting, school refusal, and threatening behavior all may become cause for arrest, involvement with the juvenile court, and possible incarceration, rather than treatment. For some youths who have negative self-images fueled by feelings of incompetence or inadequacy, entry into the juvenile justice system may be facilitated through relationships with delinquent peers, from whom they seek acceptance. Others, whose behaviors are not amenable to parental control, may be referred to the juvenile justice system by their parents in the hope that the court will provide appropriate structure and containment. Adolescents in this condition may be labeled "beyond control," "persons in need of service (PINS)," "children in need of service (CHINS)," or similar designations. In Connecticut families with children referred to the court for statutory offenses, offenses that would not require court involvement if committed by an adult, are known as "families with service needs (FWSN)." Adolescents with findings of statutory offense who enter the court system for the purpose of behavioral control place themselves at additional risk of receiving delinquency charges if they are unable or unwilling to comply with court rulings.

Adolescents in the juvenile justice system who are appropriate candidates for IICAPS services are those who have a coexisting emotional disorder and a family willing to work to maintain the youth in the home and community. Effective services for this population are likely to require the involvement and support of the adolescent's probation officer and access to court-related services that are able to provide structure and containment if needed as part of the therapeutic IICAPS intervention. For many adolescents appropriate treatment includes preparation for independence through social and vocational skill building.

## IICAPS Treatment Plan with Attainment Scales

| Child's Name | Date of Birth | Date of Intake | Date of Treatment Plan/Review |
|---|---|---|---|
| Alex | March 1, 1997 | April 4, 2005 | |

### Main Problem(s):

*Aggressive and out of control behavior, dangerous towards self*

**How likely is this behavior to result in hospitalization?**

Attainment Scale:   1   2   3   4   5   6   7   8   9   10

     (imminent risk)    (moderate risk)     (low risk)

**Goals of Treatment:** Each goal is a brief statement in terms that indicate a positive resolution of a problem or need, as seen in a demonstrated new behavior. Goals should be determined by the family with the IICAPS team.

**Action Steps:** Assignments or tasks; means of realizing treatment goals; states how or what treatments the team will utilize to facilitate a specific change in behavior. The role responsibilities of team members should be clearly stated i.e. who will do what.

Each Attainment Scale is completed by the family with the IICAPS team. The family needs to answer the question, "How successful are we at doing a particular Action Step?" Also, "How successful are we at reaching a particular goal?" On the attainment scale, replace the word "behavior" with a concrete behavior that exemplifies this level of goal attainment e.g. "wets the bed every night"; "wets the bed once a week"; "no wetting for one month."

### I. Child Domain:

Strengths: *cute, cuddly, likes animals*

Vulnerabilities: *Alex hears voices, worries, impulsive*

Figure 6.2. Treatment Plan with Attainment Scales: Alex

**Child Goal 1:** *Alex will control his behavior.*

**How successful are we at reaching the goal?**

| Attainment Scale: | 1 | 2 | 3 | 4 | 5 | 6 | 7 | 8 | 9 | 10 |
|---|---|---|---|---|---|---|---|---|---|---|
| | (behavior) | | | | (behavior) | | | | (behavior) | |
| | No action taken | | | | | | | | completed | |

**Action Step 1.1:** *Team will work with Alex to use words to express his feelings.*

| Attainment Scale: | 1 | 2 | 3 | 4 | 5 | 6 | 7 | 8 | 9 | 10 |
|---|---|---|---|---|---|---|---|---|---|---|
| | (behavior) | | | | (behavior) | | | | (behavior) | |
| | Not at all | | | | | | | | completed | |

**Action Step 1.2:** *Team will work with Alex to learn ways to control his anger and reduce his level of stress.*

| Attainment Scale: | 1 | 2 | 3 | 4 | 5 | 6 | 7 | 8 | 9 | 10 |
|---|---|---|---|---|---|---|---|---|---|---|
| | (behavior) | | | | (behavior) | | | | (behavior) | |
| | Not at all | | | | | | | | completed | |

## II. Child and Family Domain:

Strengths: *Alex's family loves one another, family works hard to support Alex, everyone pitches in as needed*

Vulnerabilities: *Alex's father had psychiatric problems, Alex's mother feels overwhelmed*

**Family Goal 1:** *Parents will learn to help manage Alex's behavior more effectively.*

**How successful are we at reaching the goal?**

| Attainment Scale: | 1 | 2 | 3 | 4 | 5 | 6 | 7 | 8 | 9 | 10 |
|---|---|---|---|---|---|---|---|---|---|---|
| | (behavior) | | | | (behavior) | | | | (behavior) | |
| | No action taken | | | | | | | | completed | |

**Action Step 1.1:** *Alex's parents will learn how to reward his good behaviors.*

| Attainment Scale: | 1 | 2 | 3 | 4 | 5 | 6 | 7 | 8 | 9 | 10 |
|---|---|---|---|---|---|---|---|---|---|---|
| | (behavior) | | | | (behavior) | | | | (behavior) | |
| | Not at all | | | | | | | | completed | |

**Action Step 1.2:** *Alex's sisters will engage in activities outside the home.*

| Attainment Scale: | 1 | 2 | 3 | 4 | 5 | 6 | 7 | 8 | 9 | 10 |
|---|---|---|---|---|---|---|---|---|---|---|
| | (behavior) | | | | (behavior) | | | | (behavior) | |
| | Not at all | | | | | | | | | completed |

## III. Child/School Domain:

Strengths: *Alex goes to school, has some friends at school*

Vulnerabilities: *Alex is a troublemaker in class, school does not manage him well.*

**School Goal 1:** *Alex will be placed in a therapeutic school.*

**How successful are we at reaching the goal?**

| Attainment Scale: | 1 | 2 | 3 | 4 | 5 | 6 | 7 | 8 | 9 | 10 |
|---|---|---|---|---|---|---|---|---|---|---|
| | (behavior) | | | | (behavior) | | | | (behavior) | |
| | No action taken | | | | | | | | | completed |

**Action Step 1.1:** *Mother and Team will request a PPT to get Alex an appropriate school placement.*

| Attainment Scale: | 1 | 2 | 3 | 4 | 5 | 6 | 7 | 8 | 9 | 10 |
|---|---|---|---|---|---|---|---|---|---|---|
| | (behavior) | | | | (behavior) | | | | (behavior) | |
| | Not at all | | | | | | | | | completed |

## IV. Physical Environment and Other Systems Domain (including adequacy of housing, and extended support systems):

Strengths: *Family lives in good neighborhood and has a very well maintained apartment. Alex has an outpatient therapist and a psychiatrist.*

Vulnerabilities: *Alex has no planned activities during times he is not in school. Alex's sisters do not have extracurricular activities.*

**Physical Environment and Other Systems Goal 1:** *Family will discuss options for after school and weekend activities that meet their interests.*

**How successful are we at reaching the goal?**

| Attainment Scale: | 1 | 2 | 3 | 4 | 5 | 6 | 7 | 8 | 9 | 10 |
|---|---|---|---|---|---|---|---|---|---|---|
| | (behavior) | | | | (behavior) | | | | (behavior) | |
| | No action taken | | | | | | | | | completed |

**Action Step 1.1:** *Parents will identify extracurricular activities in which the children can participate.*

| Attainment Scale: | 1 | 2 | 3 | 4 | 5 | 6 | 7 | 8 | 9 | 10 |
|---|---|---|---|---|---|---|---|---|---|---|
| | (behavior) Not at all | | | | (behavior) | | | | (behavior) completed | |

## Summary of Goals (group goals by domain):

**Child:** *Alex will control his behavior.*

**Family:** *Parents will learn to help manage Alex's behavior more effectively.*

**School:** *Alex will be placed in a therapeutic school.*

**Physical Environment and Other Systems:** *Family will discuss options for after school and weekend activities that meet their interests.*

**Signatures:**

| | | |
|---|---|---|
| **Parent :**_____ | **Date:** _____ |
| **Parent :**_____ | **Date:** _____ |
| **Child   :**_____ | **Date:** _____ |
| **Clinician:**_____ | **Date:** _____ |
| **Mental Health Counselor :**_____ | **Date:** _____ |
| **Supervisor** _____ | **Date:** _____ |

## Case Illustration: Cindy

REFERRAL INFORMATION

At the time of her referral to IICAPS by her probation officer, Cindy was a 14-year-old African American girl with a history of behavioral and emotional difficulties that included reckless and dangerous behaviors. Over the past seven years, Cindy had had five psychiatric hospitalizations. The most recent of these was the precipitant for her referral to IICAPS. Cindy lived with her mother and a younger brother who was 11 years of age. Her father had died in an automobile accident five years earlier. There was a suspicion that both of Cindy's parents struggled with problems of addiction.

DIAGNOSIS

Cindy was referred for IICAPS services prior to her discharge from the hospital. Cindy was known to have made multiple suicidal gestures and to cut herself frequently. She was also sexually promiscuous. Participation in the theft of at least one automobile had resulted in her referral to the juvenile justice system, and she was currently on probation. Cindy admitted to occasionally drinking alcohol and smoking marijuana but denied regular substance use. She did not adhere regularly to prescribed medication protocols and would take her medications only when she was hospitalized or wanted to "calm down." Cindy's cognitive functioning placed her in the low average range on I.Q. testing with a clear deficit in verbal ability. Cindy was enrolled in a therapeutic school because she could not be contained in a local special education program. She attended the therapeutic school about 60 percent of the time but was often tardy and disruptive in class. The school provided therapy and medication management for her.

Cindy was discharged from the hospital with an Axis I diagnosis of Bipolar Disorder with Mixed Features and a rule/out of Conduct Disorder and Polysubstance Abuse Disorder. Her diagnosis on Axis II was Borderline Traits; on Axis III was mild Asthma and on Axis IV were Severe Environmental Stressors as a result of her involvement in the juvenile justice system and the sequelae of her father's death. Her GAF score was 38. When Cindy returned home, she was prescribed 600 milligrams of lithium carbonate twice daily and 10 milligrams of Olanzapine, an antipsychotic, at night.

THE FAMILY

Cindy was nine years old when her father was killed in an automobile accident. He had a history of Bipolar Disorder, alcoholism, and substance abuse and was allegedly intoxicated when he drove a car into oncoming traffic on the highway. This may not have been an accidental event, as he had made several previous suicide attempts.

Cindy's mother was also known to have abused illegal substances in the past. She had not used drugs in many years and had entered recovery at the time of her husband's death. While her parenting skills were considered minimally adequate, she was easily overwhelmed and stressed. She was reported to love and care about her children, but she was unable to cope with Cindy's behaviors.

Cindy's mother had a reasonably well-paying job as a receptionist in a law firm. However, her job did not cover her children's health insurance, for which she received public support. The family lived in a home inherited by Cindy's mother at the death of Cindy's grandmother.

## IICAPS Intervention

ASSESSMENT & ENGAGEMENT PHASE

Cindy's oppositional behavior was evident immediately upon her return home from the hospital. She refused to take her medication, stating that she didn't like the way the medication made her feel and she hated the side effects. When she made clear that she would not alter her stance, her mother, who wanted to avoid any conflict with her daughter, let the issue drop. During the early stages of the IICAPS intervention, Cindy refused to participate in sessions with the team. She did not participate in the creation of the Genogram, the Eco-Domain Map, or the identification of her Strengths & Vulnerabilities. However, her younger brother, who was eager to learn more about his father and to gain an understanding of his sister's behavior, was very willing to engage in the intervention.

In the initial stages of the assessment process the IICAPS team observed Cindy in her school program. She was found to be inattentive, provocative, and in constant need of redirection and limit setting. School appeared to be a social rather than an educational opportunity for her, particularly in regard to her flirtatious and teasing interactions with boys. The team arranged a meeting with Cindy's probation officer, who believed that although Cindy was on probation her delinquent behavior was secondary to her manic episodes, a presumption conveyed to the probation officer by Cindy's therapist. The therapist and the probation officer believed that Cindy's needs would be better served by the mental health system rather than through the juvenile justice system.

Through the process of team supervision and rounds, the IICAPS team began to recognize that Cindy's Bipolar Disorder was not the sole cause of her behavior. Cindy appeared to use her psychiatric diagnosis to excuse behaviors that were in fact intentional. The team faced the challenge of differentiating between behaviors that resulted from her Bipolar Disorder and those that were secondary to her character structure. Although the IICAPS team agreed that Cindy's psychiatric and family histories played a substantive role in shaping her behavior, everyone involved felt that the IICAPS intervention needed to be focused in the present.

WORK & ACTION PHASE

The Assessment & Engagement Phase ended when both the team and the family recognized that Cindy needed external controls to change her behaviors. It was highly unlikely, given her resistance to involvement in the work of IICAPS, that she would be able to make the needed changes by herself. In fact, unless she was helped to adopt a healthier level of functioning, her behaviors could necessitate placement in a residential treatment center. As Cindy continued to refuse to participate in treatment, her mother and the IICAPS team developed an initial Treatment Plan (shown in Figure 6.3 at the end of the case illustration) that they hoped would lead to improvements in her behavior. However, they also agreed that if the plan failed, they would pursue residential treatment as a last resort.

During the initial weeks of the Work & Action Phase the IICAPS team and Cindy's mother crafted a strategy to gain consensus among all the service providers working with Cindy. Although the Treatment Plan required the support of all the professionals working with Cindy, they believed that it would not be successful without the unqualified support of Cindy's therapist and her psychiatrist. As a result, Cindy's mother and the IICAPS team scheduled a meeting with both persons shortly after drafting the Treatment Plan. To their surprise the school principal had been asked by the therapist to attend the meeting. The team and Cindy's mother presented the plan and described their perception that Cindy required a strong, authoritarian approach with external controls to reduce her problematic behaviors. Cindy's mother spoke movingly of her inability to limit Cindy's behavior and her fear that Cindy's activities would result in her being injured or worse. The team and Cindy's mother suggested that an active collaboration between the school and the juvenile court might provide the level of intervention needed to prevent Cindy from further dangerous behaviors. Neither the clinicians nor the principal received these recommendations enthusiastically. They were concerned that the court might not act in the best interest of Cindy or her family.

Cindy's mother and the IICAPS team understood the concerns. However, given what appeared to be Cindy's elevated risk for potential danger, they believed that the active involvement of the juvenile court was the least detrimental alternative for her. During this meeting, Cindy's mother and the team reiterated the need for consensus among all the providers, including the probation officer and the court. Within several days, the school therapist and the principal agreed to the recommendations. Their agreement may have been influenced by Cindy's increasingly disruptive and sexualized behaviors at school.

The plan proposed by the team and Cindy's mother quickly received the support of Cindy's probation officer and her supervisor. Within a short time a court hearing was held, and Cindy was ordered by the judge to obey a 6:00 P.M. curfew daily and to comply with all aspects of her treatment. In addition, Cindy was referred to a partial hospital program so that her behaviors could be more closely monitored.

At her court appearance, Cindy agreed to comply with the judge's orders. However, the following day she stayed out until 10:30 P.M., violating her curfew. Her mother responded by reporting her behavior to the probation officer. Cindy's noncompliant behavior continued for more than a week. She refused to meet with the IICAPS team, continued to disregard her curfew, and did not attend a scheduled appointment with her psychiatrist. She did keep her intake appointment with staff of the partial hospital.

At this point in the work, the IICAPS team urged her probation officer to place Cindy on house arrest with an electronic monitor. Cindy was allowed to leave the house only to attend school and partial hospital. Although Cindy continued to be noncompliant with her medication, she complied with her house arrest for approximately one week. Shortly thereafter, she cut the ankle bracelet that served as the electronic monitor, left home, and did not return. Cindy was picked up by police three days after running away and was brought to the detention center on a court order. Cindy's behavior was not unexpected. In anticipation, the provider group had already made plans that could be put into place if such behavior occurred. Within three days of her detainment, Cindy was rehospitalized. At the time of her hospital admission, a request was made to commit her to her mother's care so that she could be properly medicated. Within five days of admission to the hospital

Cindy was started on a long-acting intramuscular antipsychotic medication. In response, her impulsivity, rage, and mania decreased markedly. She was discharged from the hospital within seven days with follow-up plans in place. She continued on electronically monitored house arrest for three weeks and was compliant with court orders after the monitoring was removed.

ENDING & WRAP-UP PHASE

Once Cindy's behaviors stabilized and her mother was able to manage her behaviors reasonably well, the IICAPS intervention entered the Ending & Wrap-Up Phase. Although Cindy continued to have some difficulties at school and was not fully engaged in therapy, her mother felt that she had her daughter back. One of the remaining tasks of this phase was to advocate for the extension of both Cindy's probation for an additional six months and her weekly monitoring by her probation officer.

While Cindy refused to comply with recommendations that she take a mood stabilizer and continued to test limits, she did agree to attend regular psychiatric and medical appointments and to use birth control. Although there were still issues that could have been addressed as part of the IICAPS intervention, Cindy's mother felt that after eight months of working with the team, the family was as stable as it was going to be. In accordance with IICAPS principles, Cindy would continue her treatment with her outpatient providers now that the need for intensive in-home intervention had lessened. In addition to Cindy's individual treatment and medication management, Cindy and her mother agreed to participate in weekly family therapy sessions. If the need arose, another referral could be made for additional IICAPS intervention.

## IICAPS Treatment Plan with Attainment Scales

| Child's Name | Date of Birth | Date of Intake | Date of Treatment Plan/Review |
|---|---|---|---|
| Cindy | June 21, 1990 | November 17, 2004 | |

### Main Problem(s):

*Aggressive and dangerous behavior primarily at home*

**How likely is this behavior to result in hospitalization?**

Attainment Scale:  1     2     3     4     5     6     7     8     9     10
                  (imminent risk)          (moderate risk)          (low risk)

**Goals of Treatment:** Each goal is a brief statement in terms that indicate a positive resolution of a problem or need, as seen in a demonstrated new behavior. Goals should be determined by the family with the IICAPS team.

**Action Steps:** Assignments or tasks; means of realizing treatment goals; states how or what treatments the team will utilize to facilitate a specific change in behavior. The role responsibilities of team members should be clearly stated i.e. who will do what.

Each Attainment Scale is completed by the family with the IICAPS team. The family needs to answer the question, "How successful are we at doing a particular Action Step?" Also, "How successful are we at reaching a particular goal?" On the attainment scale, replace the word "behavior" with a concrete behavior that exemplifies this level of goal attainment e.g. "wets the bed every night"; "wets the bed once a week"; "no wetting for one month."

### I. Child Domain:

Strengths: *Attractive, good sense of humor*

Vulnerabilities: *Refuses to participate in treatment, lies, steals, impulsive*

Figure 6.3. Initial Treatment Plan: Cindy

**Child Goal 1:** *Cindy will be medication compliant.*

**How successful are we at reaching the goal?**

| Attainment Scale: | 1 | 2 | 3 | 4 | 5 | 6 | 7 | 8 | 9 | 10 |
|---|---|---|---|---|---|---|---|---|---|---|
| | (behavior) | | | | (behavior) | | | | (behavior) | |
| | No action taken | | | | | | | | completed | |

**Action Step 1.1:** *IICAPS team with Cindy's mother will work with other providers to seek support from juvenile probation to create consequences through the court process for her behavior.*

| Attainment Scale: | 1 | 2 | 3 | 4 | 5 | 6 | 7 | 8 | 9 | 10 |
|---|---|---|---|---|---|---|---|---|---|---|
| | (behavior) | | | | (behavior) | | | | (behavior) | |
| | Not at all | | | | | | | | completed | |

**Action Step 1.2:** *Cindy will be informed of plan after meeting with juvenile probation officer and that medication adherence is an essential part of plan.*

| Attainment Scale: | 1 | 2 | 3 | 4 | 5 | 6 | 7 | 8 | 9 | 10 |
|---|---|---|---|---|---|---|---|---|---|---|
| | (behavior) | | | | (behavior) | | | | (behavior) | |
| | Not at all | | | | | | | | completed | |

**Action Step 1.3:** *Cindy will meet regularly with her psychiatrist.*

| Attainment Scale: | 1 | 2 | 3 | 4 | 5 | 6 | 7 | 8 | 9 | 10 |
|---|---|---|---|---|---|---|---|---|---|---|
| | (behavior) | | | | (behavior) | | | | (behavior) | |
| | Not at all | | | | | | | | completed | |

**Child Goal 2:** *Cindy will participate actively in psychotherapy.*

**How successful are we at reaching the goal?**

| Attainment Scale: | 1 | 2 | 3 | 4 | 5 | 6 | 7 | 8 | 9 | 10 |
|---|---|---|---|---|---|---|---|---|---|---|
| | (behavior) | | | | (behavior) | | | | (behavior) | |
| | No action taken | | | | | | | | completed | |

**Action Step 2.1:** *IICAPS team with Cindy's mother will work with juvenile probation to create consequences through the court process for her behavior.*

| Attainment Scale: | 1 | 2 | 3 | 4 | 5 | 6 | 7 | 8 | 9 | 10 |
|---|---|---|---|---|---|---|---|---|---|---|
| | (behavior) | | | | (behavior) | | | | (behavior) | |
| | Not at all | | | | | | | | completed | |

**Action Step 2.2:** *Cindy will be informed that participation in psychotherapy is part of her court ordered plan after meeting with probation officer.*

| Attainment Scale: | 1 | 2 | 3 | 4 | 5 | 6 | 7 | 8 | 9 | 10 |
|---|---|---|---|---|---|---|---|---|---|---|
| | (behavior) | | | | (behavior) | | | | (behavior) | |
| | Not at all | | | | | | | | | completed |

**Action Step 2.3:** *Cindy will meet, at minimum, weekly with her therapist.*

| Attainment Scale: | 1 | 2 | 3 | 4 | 5 | 6 | 7 | 8 | 9 | 10 |
|---|---|---|---|---|---|---|---|---|---|---|
| | (behavior) | | | | (behavior) | | | | (behavior) | |
| | Not at all | | | | | | | | | completed |

## II. Child and Family Domain:

Strengths: *Cindy's mother cares about her, she has refrained from substance abuse, Cindy's brother is doing well in all domains*

Vulnerabilities: *Cindy's mother feels helpless in caring for Cindy*

**Family Goal 1:** *Mother will become more active in getting Cindy the treatment, support and structure that she requires.*

### How successful are we at reaching the goal?

| Attainment Scale: | 1 | 2 | 3 | 4 | 5 | 6 | 7 | 8 | 9 | 10 |
|---|---|---|---|---|---|---|---|---|---|---|
| | (behavior) | | | | (behavior) | | | | (behavior) | |
| | No action taken | | | | | | | | | completed |

**Action Step 1.1:** *Cindy's mother and Ms. Williams will meet weekly to make plans and implement them around Cindy's treatment.*

| Attainment Scale: | 1 | 2 | 3 | 4 | 5 | 6 | 7 | 8 | 9 | 10 |
|---|---|---|---|---|---|---|---|---|---|---|
| | (behavior) | | | | (behavior) | | | | (behavior) | |
| | Not at all | | | | | | | | | completed |

**Action Step 1.2:** *Cindy's mother will actively participate in meetings with Cindy's therapist, psychiatrist and probation officer.*

| Attainment Scale: | 1 | 2 | 3 | 4 | 5 | 6 | 7 | 8 | 9 | 10 |
|---|---|---|---|---|---|---|---|---|---|---|
| | (behavior) | | | | (behavior) | | | | (behavior) | |
| | Not at all | | | | | | | | | completed |

## III. Child/School Domain:

Strengths: *Cindy goes to school regularly; she is in a therapeutic school.*

Vulnerabilities: *Cindy is disruptive in class, does not do any work.*

**School Goal 1:** *Cindy will improve behavior and do school work.*

**How successful are we at reaching the goal?**

| Attainment Scale: | 1 | 2 | 3 | 4 | 5 | 6 | 7 | 8 | 9 | 10 |
|---|---|---|---|---|---|---|---|---|---|---|
| | (behavior) | | | | (behavior) | | | | (behavior) | |
| | No action taken | | | | | | | | | completed |

**Action Step 1.1:** *Mother and IICAPS teams will work with school to be part of plan with probation.*

| Attainment Scale: | 1 | 2 | 3 | 4 | 5 | 6 | 7 | 8 | 9 | 10 |
|---|---|---|---|---|---|---|---|---|---|---|
| | (behavior) | | | | (behavior) | | | | (behavior) | |
| | Not at all | | | | | | | | | completed |

## IV. Physical Environment and Other Systems Domain (including adequacy of housing, and extended support systems):

Strengths: *Family lives in safe neighborhood and has nice house; Cindy has both a therapist and a psychiatrist.*

Vulnerabilities: *Cindy does not attend therapy or medication sessions regularly.*

**Physical Environment and Other Systems Goal 1:** *Team and mother will meet with treaters to create probation plan.*

**How successful are we at reaching the goal?**

| Attainment Scale: | 1 | 2 | 3 | 4 | 5 | 6 | 7 | 8 | 9 | 10 |
|---|---|---|---|---|---|---|---|---|---|---|
| | (behavior) | | | | (behavior) | | | | (behavior) | |
| | No action taken | | | | | | | | | completed |

**Action Step1.1:** *IICAPS team with Cindy's mother will work with other providers to seek support from juvenile probation to create consequences through the court process for her behavior.*

| Attainment Scale: | 1 | 2 | 3 | 4 | 5 | 6 | 7 | 8 | 9 | 10 |
|---|---|---|---|---|---|---|---|---|---|---|
| | (behavior) | | | | (behavior) | | | | (behavior) | |
| | Not at all | | | | | | | | | completed |

**Summary of Goals (group goals by domain):**

**Child:** *Cindy will be medication compliant.  Cindy will participate actively in psychotherapy.*

**Family:** *Mother will become more active in getting Cindy the treatment, support and structure that she requires.*

**School:** *Cindy will improve behavior and do school work.*

**Physical Environment and Other Systems:** *Team and mother will meet with treaters to create probation plan.*

**Signatures:**

Parent :_____     Date: _____
Parent :_____     Date: _____
Child  :_____     Date: _____
Clinician:_____     Date: _____
Mental Health Counselor :_____     Date: _____
Supervisor _____     Date: _____

# Chapter 7 Organizational Structure

The organizational structure and practice of IICAPS are designed to reinforce the principles of integration, connectivity, and multilayered interaction that are essential elements of IICAPS programs. This chapter outlines the roles and qualifications of clinical and administrative personnel and the systemic and fiscal collaborations necessary for developing and sustaining an effective replication of the model. In the IICAPS model these disparate elements are united to form a coherent functional support mechanism for all IICAPS interventions.

An administrative team composed of a medical director, a program director, and a program coordinator, and teams of licensed or license-eligible clinicians and mental health counselors constitute the core of the intervention. The administrative support staff of the agency in which IICAPS is embedded is responsible for IICAPS business and clerical functions.

At the heart of the organizational design is a commitment to the same levels of collaboration that are expected to exist between IICAPS clinicians and the children and families with whom they work. Collaborations between administrative and clinical staff, between managers and the purchasers of services, between the private IICAPS providers and the public child mental health system, and between geographically specific IICAPS providers and IICAPS Services are central to the success of the IICAPS mission. These relationships facilitate the progress of the individual treatments, promote the stability and sustainability of the program over time, and increase the program's potential to function more broadly as a change agent in the children's mental health system.

All IICAPS programs are required to adopt an organizational structure that prescribes the qualifications, duties, and responsibilities of clinical staff, supervisors, and program managers. IICAPS programs are not expected to be free-standing; they are most likely to exist within licensed mental health agencies that also offer outpatient, school-based, and other treatment services to children and families. It is possible that in some settings, IICAPS will take its place along a continuum that also includes in-patient and residential care and other intensive in-home services such as multisystemic therapy (MST). To qualify as an IICAPS site, a program must demonstrate adherence to the organizational structure described below.

The organization of an IICAPS program is comprised of three primary, interrelated elements: a clinical team, a supervisory team, and an administrative team. At any given time, individuals working in an IICAPS program may function in one or all of these areas. In parallel with all IICAPS clinical interventions, the interrelationship between each of these organizational elements must be marked by openness and transparency. Communication between the elements must be regular, frequent, and of sufficient duration to allow for the informed and frank discussions that will propel the program forward. The development of mutual trust, professional respect, and acceptance of differences in training and orientation that are hallmarks of IICAPS are essential to the success of this process.

### CLINICAL TEAM

All children and families receiving IICAPS services are assigned to an IICAPS team that is specifically trained and supervised to provide the intervention in adherence with the treatment model. Each IICAPS team is composed of a master's-prepared clinician and a bachelor's-level mental health counselor. Each individual treatment team is embedded in the broader IICAPS organizational structure and participates in the prescribed activities that support the intervention, including weekly supervision, rounds, and program meetings.

Although training in the IICAPS model is required of all staff prior to their taking part in any clinical encounters within an IICAPS program, clinicians are expected to possess sufficient clinical knowledge and skill to perform the tasks and services demanded by the intervention at the time they become staff members. The individuals best suited to serve as mental health counselors hold bachelor's degrees with some coursework in the social sciences and are either seeking field experience before entering graduate programs or are "natural helpers" with the requisite empathy, understanding, and life experience to qualify for this work. The diverse professional and personal experiences that are desirable attributes of team members add to the richness of the treatment and assure that services are grounded in the reality of the children and families being served. The work of well-functioning teams is enhanced by the integration of each team member's individual perceptions of the family and enriched by their different viewpoints.

The support that team members provide for each other in what can be isolative, stressful, and frustrating work is among the many benefits of a team approach. Another important benefit of the team structure is the reduction in staff burnout. The ability of team members to share the crises, frustrations, and successes of doing this work contributes to greater job satisfaction and overall productivity levels. In addition, working as part of a team may increase longevity in the position as well. The team structure reinforces the interactive, multilevel IICAPS approach and serves to model partnership, co-ordination, compromise, and negotiation for children and families.

The services offered by each treatment team include individual psychotherapy, family therapy, parent guidance, behavioral management, crisis response, medication monitoring, and case management. Although the utilization of specific treatment modalities is dependent upon the need of each individual child and family, each team is expected to demonstrate the capacity to offer or access the range of interventions that may be required as part of an individual Treatment Plan.

### The Mental Health Clinician

All IICAPS clinicians are expected to possess a master's degree in social work, psychology, nursing, or a related clinical field and be licensed or license-eligible. Because IICAPS interventions have the unique capacity to address the psychological and behavioral needs of both children and adults simultaneously, individuals who qualify as IICAPS clinicians should demonstrate a thorough knowledge of child and adult development, have a working knowledge of the theories and methodologies upon which IICAPS is based, and be experienced in providing individual, group, and family psychosocial assessment and treatment. In addition, IICAPS clinicians are expected to possess innovative problem-solving, advanced crisis intervention, and management skills, as well as proficiency in oral and written communication.

Responsibilities of an IICAPS clinician are phase dependent. During the Assessment & Engagement Phase of the intervention, the clinician works in partnership with the family to collect information that will inform the assessment and evaluation of both the child's and the family's needs. With the family as a full partner, the clinician reviews the family history, in the context of the presenting problem that led to the referral for IICAPS services, using a three-generational Genogram as the primary Tool. Together they identify the family strengths and challenges and the current level of child, parent, and family functioning. The clinician guides the family in articulating the Main Problem that places the child at risk of more restrictive intervention, using the identified Strengths & Vulnerabilities to construct an Eco-Domain Map, which in turn informs the setting of the family's treatment Goals and strategies for action.

During the Work & Action Phase the clinician, in partnership with the family, the mental health counselor, the supervisor, and the rounds team, continuously reevaluates the Treatment Plan, reviews progress toward the stated Goals, and makes recommendations for any needed adjustments. During the Ending & Wrap-Up Phase, the family and the IICAPS team, including the supervisor and rounds teams, establish the criteria for discharge, develop the plan for services beyond active IICAPS intervention, and assist with the transition to the next level of care. Throughout the intervention, the clinical team and the family work in partnership to maintain the direction of the intervention and measure progress toward the Goals they have established.

The clinician is responsible for completing intake and assessment reports within three weeks of the initial intake session, maintaining required documentation of client condition and progress throughout the intervention, assuring that records are maintained in compliance with regulatory and departmental standards, and completing the mandatory discharge summary in a timely fashion.

### The Mental Health Counselor

To qualify as an IICAPS mental health counselor an individual is expected to possess either a bachelor's degree in a related field with an interest in continuing in the human service field or an associate's degree with four years of related work experience. Mental health counselors who have prior work experience should be familiar with a range of community-based services, particularly those related to the social service, health, and public welfare systems.

The clinician and the mental health counselor constitute the IICAPS treatment team. IICAPS mental health counselors provide both concrete services and emotional support to families and assist their clinician partners in assessment and service planning. The team meets with the clinical supervisor weekly to review the progress of each case. The use of the IICAPS treatment Tools and Forms assures the team's adherence to the treatment model. Tasks that are often the primary responsibility of the mental health counselor include acting as an advocate for the family with other community and social systems (for example, public assistance, housing, medical and/or mental health, education, and juvenile justice); providing parent education and guidance in specific areas (for example, basic childcare, limit setting, and behavioral management); providing concrete services (for example, transportation, accessing food banks, budgeting); and linking the family to extended family members, appropriate community resources, and social supports.

The mental health counselor works with the clinician in the assessment and treatment planning process. The mental health counselor assists in gathering the information needed by the team in the initial Phases of their work, including the history and nature of the presenting problem, the identification of the Main Problem that places the child at risk of more restrictive placement, and the description of the child's and family's needs. The mental health counselor and the clinician work with the family to recognize family stressors, strengths, and challenges and the current level of child, parental, and family functioning. In some instances, the mental health counselor is able to contribute a working knowledge of the community and to communicate effectively with family members in a manner that promotes the engagement process and facilitates the work of assessment.

The specific tasks undertaken by either the mental health counselor or the clinician will vary from case to case, depending upon the nature of the treatment alliance that develops between the child, the family, and the two team members. As a result, at some times the licensed clinician may conduct family or child sessions with the mental health counselor in attendance; at other times, each may act independently. When the work demands, both members of the team may be present for an encounter though focused on separate tasks. Together with the family, the clinician, the mental health counselor, and the

IICAPS supervisor continuously reassess the methods by which the work will be accomplished. Through this process they address the specific tasks they have identified and update the Treatment Plan in accordance with the family's progress toward its Goals. The multilevel involvement that characterizes the IICAPS approach supports contributions of peers, program coordinators, and medical directors to the process of continuous Treatment Plan review and modification. IICAPS places high value on the sharing of clinical knowledge and resource information and encourages team members to ask for and receive assistance when they are uncertain about any aspect of the work.

### Shared Characteristics of Team Members

Clinicians and the mental health counselors are expected to have differing academic and professional training and to carry specific, complementary responsibilities within the treatment team. However, both members of the team should possess the qualities and characteristics that are vital for successful IICAPS interventions. Essential attributes for team members include patience and flexibility, the ability to be accepting of individual differences, and the willingness to recognize and accommodate families' needs, rather than make a priori assumptions about these needs. Of equal importance is the capacity to accept and respect each family's history, culture, value preferences, and lifestyles. Both members of the team should be good observers and good listeners, who are comfortable setting appropriate limits and able to work together to handle unexpected situations and crises as they arise. Experience working with children with serious emotional disturbances and their families, the willingness to work in the child's home and not in a traditional clinic setting, a sense of personal boundaries, strong ethics, and mature judgment are all prerequisites for IICAPS team members. Nevertheless, team members should also be comfortable asking for supervision and consultation whenever needed. In appreciation of the challenges inherent in this work, IICAPS is purposefully structured to facilitate access to supervision. Clinicians and mental health counselors are supervised as a team; both members of the team are required to attend weekly rounds, supervisory sessions, and program meetings. In addition, clinical consultation and support are accessible at all levels of involvement and at all times of day or night through beeper and on-call rotation.

### Supervision

The IICAPS model provides for two interrelated levels of supervision, each designed to expand the context and understanding of the therapeutic work while providing guidance and stimulation for team members. The chaos and disorganization that characterize the lives of many IICAPS families call for focused intervention. Because it is essential that IICAPS Treatment Plans identify manageable problems that are amenable to focused solutions, those engaged in doing the work must be aided and supported in thinking in unorthodox ways. Although the intervention does make use of traditional assessments and treatment strategies, team members are encouraged to think creatively and to adapt their interventions to the specific needs and characteristics of each child and family. IICAPS supervisors, like all other IICAPS staff members, must be trained formally in the IICAPS model. Supervisors are required to use IICAPS Tools and Forms to perform the multiple tasks for which they have been designed: engagement, assessment, intervention, quality assurance, and supervision. Familiarity with the Concepts, Tools, and Forms that guide progress through the IICAPS Phases and Domains provides structure and guidance for supervisors. At the same time, use of the Tools promotes and assures fidelity to the IICAPS model.

The supervisor plays an important role in the process of applying theoretical constructs and evidence-based knowledge to the work of the team while also leading them to think creatively. Supervisors should be knowledgeable about key tenets of developmental psychopathology, family therapy, psychoanalytic theory, and cognitive-behavioral interventions and comfortable with their application.

Although all IICAPS supervisors must have prior experience supervising clinicians in a mental health setting, they continue to be supervised in this role by the child and adolescent psychiatrist, who as medical director of the IICAPS program is also a consultant and advisor to the supervisor. IICAPS supervisors are expected to attend rounds regularly and to serve as members of the site-specific management team. Most commonly the supervisor acts as the IICAPS program coordinator and assumes both clinical and administrative responsibilities.

In addition to regular weekly team-specific supervision, teams are required to present each of their cases for group discussion and review every three weeks at clinical rounds that are held weekly and also attended by supervisors. Rounds are co-led by the IICAPS medical director and the program coordinator. Others in regular attendance are all other clinicians and mental health counselor teams in the particular program, and the liaison from the public mental health agency. Rounds presentations are governed by IICAPS rounds protocols and schedules, which are discussed fully in Chapter 8. IICAPS tools, including the Genogram, the Eco-Domain Map, and the Treatment Plan with Goal Attainment Scales, are presented at prescribed intervals. Rounds provide another opportunity to measure adherence to the model.

## Program Coordinator

### CLINICAL ROLE

IICAPS program coordinators manage the day-to-day functioning of the program and frequently play both clinical and administrative roles. An IICAPS program coordinator must have a master's or doctoral degree in psychology, social work, or nursing and be in possession of an active state license to provide mental health services. The IICAPS model supports the program coordinator's active participation as a member of an IICAPS clinical team. By spending a portion of time working in the field as an IICAPS clinician, the program coordinator gains important firsthand knowledge of the challenges, concerns, and opportunities faced regularly by IICAPS teams that can be used to inform effective supervision and administration.

### ADMINISTRATIVE ROLE

The program coordinator is responsible for handling intake and referrals for the IICAPS program, determining if the child and family meet the eligibility criteria for service, making clinical team and supervisory assignments, monitoring case flow, scheduling rounds presentations, managing the waiting list, training staff in administrative procedures, assuring that patient charts are maintained in timely fashion, monitoring billing and insurance authorizations, and facilitating weekly staff meetings. As a member of the IICAPS administrative team, the program coordinator participates in all aspects of program management, functions as a liaison between the administrative team and the clinical staff, and represents the program in dealing with the other local community agencies with which it interacts when appropriate.

### ADMINISTRATIVE TEAM

The persistent attention to the complex human interrelationships that characterizes all IICAPS clinical care is reflected in the composition and function of the IICAPS administrative team, a required structural element of IICAPS programs. Just as the needs and demands of the child and the family are affected by the dynamic interactions between them, so, too, the quality and nature of the clinical work are affected by the relationships between the clinical team, the supervisors, and the senior managers of the program. The IICAPS administrative team is intended to function as the vehicle through which positive interactions at all levels of the programs are promoted, conflicts resolved, and a supportive and growth-promoting environment sustained. Clinical work across both traditional outpatient and in-patient settings is influenced by the quality of the work environment and the amount of support provided for individual clinicians. However, the degree of intimacy demanded of clinicians who work exclusively in a home setting requires an organization structure that mediates stress and allows for positive, open, honest, and noncompetitive interaction among all members of the organization.

The administrative team is composed of the IICAPS medical director, the program director, and the program coordinator. Each member of the team is involved in the primary operation of the program and able to exercise considerable influence over its functioning. The prescribed weekly meeting of the IICAPS administrative team provides a regular opportunity to discuss and resolve issues involving staff, program development, and ongoing training, to monitor adherence to the IICAPS model, and to address managerial and fiscal matters.

Each member of the administrative team bears a specific set of program responsibilities. The ultimate effectiveness of the program is dependent upon the degree to which the various program elements come together to form a coherent and seamless whole. The ability of the team to grapple with the tensions and strains of administering IICAPS services will have a profound and direct influence on the outcomes of the individual case interventions. At the discretion of the program director, the administrative team may be augmented by the participation of others who are involved at a senior level of program management and/or supervision of IICAPS clinical teams.

### Medical Director

All IICAPS programs are required to conform to a specific model of medical and programmatic administration that reinforces their commitment to the provision of mental health services of the highest quality. The administrative structure of IICAPS programs supports the duality of the IICAPS mission: to maintain children with serious psychiatric conditions safely in the least restrictive environments possible and to act as a mental health systems change agent. For decades, child and adolescent psychiatrists, the most highly trained professionals concerned with the care of children with serious mental health disorders, have been distanced from community mental health systems. The complicated array of factors that led to the isolation of the child psychiatrist from those with regular professional involvement with children, including teachers, probation officers, and other mental health workers, was described in Chapter 1. In contradistinction to the view that the role of the child psychiatrist is primarily that of prescriber and manager of medication, the IICAPS model supports the presumption that the potential long-term effects of the debilitating level of psychopathology currently found among children, adolescents, and their families can be addressed most efficiently and economically through consistent utilization of the training and skills of child psychiatrists. Reflecting support of this belief, the medical director of an IICAPS program must be a board-certified child and adolescent psychiatrist.

The medical director of an IICAPS program has medico-legal responsibility for the clinical care of all the children served by the program. Before accepting this level of responsibility, medical directors are required to participate in IICAPS training to become familiar with the IICAPS model, including theory, implementation strategies, rounds processes, tools, and required documentation. The prescribed clinical responsibilities of the medical director are to conduct weekly program rounds at which cases are presented according to specific rounds protocols and which provide important teaching opportunities, to act as a consultant to program supervisors and members of the clinical teams, to serve as a team supervisor when contracted to do so, and to perform medication assessments and monitoring when appropriate for children in the program.

The administrative responsibilities of the medical director include serving as a full member of the management team, participating in staff training at the request of the program director or coordinator, and attending multisite IICAPS Network meetings, some of which are for medical directors exclusively. The medical director may be called upon to act as an essential intermediary in the process of negotiating between managed-care entities and the IICAPS program and articulating the factors that satisfy the medical-necessity criteria for reimbursement. The medical director is expected to be a strong advocate for the mental health services needed by children in the IICAPS program.

Once an IICAPS program expands to a caseload of 35 children and families or more, it is no longer possible for the IICAPS rounds schedule to be maintained in the prescribed order of rotation and recommended presentation time. Programs that serve 36 or more children and families are required to develop a second rounds team and to enlist the services of an additional child and adolescent psychiatrist to serve on the IICAPS staff as the leader of the new team. It is expected that the staff child psychiatrist will also be available for individual team supervision and consultation when needed and will perform psychiatric and medication assessments and monitoring as appropriate for children in the program.

### Program Director

Because IICAPS programs are not designed to be free-standing entities, they are most likely to be embedded in larger mental health organizations such as child guidance clinics or social service agencies, whose missions resonate with that of IICAPS. Just as the fit between the child, the family, and the IICAPS clinical team is thought to be a critical element in a successful intervention, the fit between the parent organization and the IICAPS program is strongly correlated with the program's development, maintenance, and sustainability. The link between the IICAPS program and the parent organization is the program director, a senior staff person with a high level of responsibility and decision-making capability. The program director provides leadership for the program, acts as the primary program administrator, represents the program both within and outside the parent organization, and has overall responsibility for its implementation. The scope of the program director's responsibilities is broad, ranging from the integration of the IICAPS program into the structure and clinical goals of the parent organization to the establishment of a program-specific work environment that supports a staff that is subject regularly to the stressors arising from the frequent clinical challenges and frustrations that emerge from the work. The program director is expected to balance the clinical, political, and fiscal demands that characterize the mental health system of the twenty-first century.

The program director has overall responsibility for the implementation and management of the IICAPS program and its adherence to the IICAPS model (for example, hiring, referral processes, charting, recordkeeping, administration of measures, and treatment planning). The program director participates in the development of contracts, grants, and additional sources of funding and monitors all data submission and compliance with requests for reports or other information. The program director may act as a clinical supervisor for an IICAPS team, and is expected to provide case consultation as needed, attend weekly rounds, and serve as a member of the management team.

The program director and the program coordinator represent the IICAPS program in all communication between the program and the IICAPS Services

Network. In addition, the program director, with other staff, represents the program in the community and advocates on its behalf. The program director should hold a master's or doctoral degree in psychology, social work, public health, or a related field and have experience in the development, implementation, and management of clinical programs for children with serious emotional disturbances and their families.

## PARENTS/CAREGIVERS

Parents provide the family setting in which the majority of the IICAPS intervention takes place. The venue symbolizes the shift in control inherent in the IICAPS model. Each interaction between the team and the family should be characterized by respect and acceptance. Parents or other adults acting as primary caregivers are expected to play essential roles as full partners in the intervention. Working with the team, they take the lead in identifying the primary issues to be addressed, setting the Goals of the treatment, and participating actively in all aspects of the service. Because family members are expected to be the primary care providers for their child following the IICAPS intervention, it is essential that they "buy in" to the work, understand its purpose, acknowledge the need for change, and exhibit an interest in bringing change about. As a voluntary service, IICAPS is dependent for its implementation upon the parents' willingness to work with the clinical team. However, the process of engaging parents as active collaborators and members of the broader intervention team may vary significantly from case to case. The ultimate goal of the first Phase of the intervention is to actualize the partnership through the building of a trusting relationship between the family and the team. It is this alliance that enables the work to move forward to the point that the child and family can function without the services of the clinical team.

## PUBLIC MENTAL HEALTH
## AGENCY REPRESENTATIVE

Each IICAPS program should have one high-level public child mental health agency liaison who attends weekly rounds, the opportunity for clinical case review. The overarching purpose of the liaison position is to assure appropriate and timely coordination of services for children who are involved with the public mental health agency while they are receiving IICAPS services. The primary task of the individual serving as liaison is to facilitate treatment planning and implementation. When there is an issue involving the public agency, the liaison is expected to convey information that is presented by IICAPS teams at rounds to the public agency staff members who are involved in the case. In addition, the liaison is able to provide ongoing training and consultation to the treatment teams concerning relevant publicly funded programs, policies, and personnel to facilitate treatment.

## COMMUNITY PROVIDERS AND SYSTEMS

The multilayered IICAPS approach incorporates a network of family and community partners into each child's Treatment Plan. The active involvement of case-specific extended family members, such as grandparents; community-based care providers, the child's outpatient therapist and primary health care provider; and representatives of the systems in which the child is involved, such as school and protective services, ensures case coordination and service integration. Facilitated by the IICAPS clinical team, regularly scheduled case-specific meetings bring these individuals together for purposes of goal setting, treatment planning, and implementation. Some members of this group may continue working with the child and family well beyond the time of the intervention itself. Although individual and family change is the goal of the intervention, systems change often occurs as an important by-product of the intervention.

## ADMINISTRATIVE SUPPORT

The successful implementation of a program requires the efforts of a support team composed of administrative assistants and business staff. Administrative assistants should have good interpersonal skills, as they can be expected to interact with families on the telephone, demonstrate patience and professionalism regarding client confidentiality, and be good listeners. Specific tasks include computerized data management, updating patient records, submitting reports, maintaining case files, and providing such clerical support and assistance as needed by the program director, coordinator, and staff. The business office handles budgetary issues, monitors collections against claims and costs, supervises and assists with grant work, and disperses payroll to staff.

## IICAPS SERVICES

All IICAPS programs in Connecticut are part of the IICAPS Services Network. The Network is facilitated and staffed by the program developers and their representatives as part of IICAPS Services, the training and data collection arm of the model. IICAPS Services staff provide the training in the IICAPS model, which is required for all teams, medical directors, supervisors, and administrators. Before assuming any position in the IICAPS system, individuals are required to attend 15 hours of manualized training sessions through which they become familiar with the basic IICAPS elements. These sessions are offered monthly; booster sessions for experienced staff are offered quarterly.

IICAPS Services staff engage in monthly consultation with the IICAPS site directors, medical directors, and coordinators to review issues emanating from the work and to discuss clinical as well as administrative problems. In addition to scheduled monthly case-focused consultations, program supervisors are invited to participate in monthly telephone conference calls that address issues specific to supervising home-based treatment using the IICAPS model. All site directors, coordinators, and supervisors may request additional site-specific information or consultation from IICAPS Services at any time.

IICAPS Services facilitates quarterly meetings for teams, coordinators, supervisors, and public agency liaisons. The meetings provide an opportunity for ongoing training on clinical topics relevant to the work as well as open discussion of the issues related to implementation of the model. The IICAPS Services also facilitates a quarterly meeting for leadership of IICAPS sites. These meetings are more intimate than the larger Network meeting and focus upon issues of supervision, management, protocols, funding, and the like. Because IICAPS Services serves as the data collection arm for all IICAPS programs for the Connecticut Department of Children and Families, the initial funder of the model and one of its strongest supporters, the meetings also offer an opportunity to provide feedback from the continuous data collection and data analysis efforts.

The development of the Network and the facilitation of the leadership meetings are important components of the IICAPS strategy for systems change. IICAPS has created a venue in which providers and public agency staff are able to regularly discuss the ways in which the application of key concepts and principles of developmental psychopathology can be applied broadly to improve the treatment of the many children with SED.

# Chapter 8 Quality Assurance

## SUPERVISION: AN IICAPS
## FIDELITY MEASURE

Supervision is a central element of the IICAPS model. The paramount objective of supervision in the IICAPS model is to provide an effective, replicable quality-assurance/improvement process. To accomplish this goal, supervision is expected to facilitate each clinician's acquisition and implementation of the clinical skills required by IICAPS and consistent with the specific components of the IICAPS Fidelity Mechanisms: Principles, Concepts, and Tools. The clinical skills of IICAPS team members are critical to the attenuation or elimination of the identified Main Problem and the achievement of positive, sustainable outcomes. Supervision is the process by which a senior mental health clinician helps team members to optimize treatment using the structure of the IICAPS case-specific Fidelity Mechanisms. The methodology used to create these mechanisms follows closely the supervision techniques defined by Henggeler and used in multisystemic therapy (Henggeler et al., 1998).

IICAPS supervision occurs in two venues: clinical supervision and rounds. The primary function of IICAPS clinical supervision and rounds is to ensure that clinicians are able, on a consistent basis, to utilize the IICAPS Principles, Concepts, and Tools in all aspects of treatment planning, implementation, and refinement.

### Guidelines for Supervisors

The challenges and opportunities that occur during supervision mirror those of treatment. For this reason, the guidelines for supervision (see Table 8.1) are consistent with the IICAPS treatment principles. Supervisor adherence is monitored through self-reports, data submission, and consultant evaluation.

The supervisory relationship provides the critical context of clinical support for the clinical team and is the pivotal factor in shaping the treatment process (Lindblad-Goldberg, Dore, and Stern, 1998). Looking at the ongoing processes of treatment, the supervisor must help the clinical team remain a neutral consultant to the family and devise effective approaches to the work. Operating from a more objective perspective, the supervisor helps the clinical team maintain accountability during the intervention. This process is an attempt to ensure fidelity to the model by consistently monitoring the team's adherence to IICAPS Principles, Concepts, and Tools. Believing that the clinical team can be held accountable for its behavior and still continue to grow professionally and personally, the supervisor assesses and informs the clinical team's work, both to better meet the needs of children and families and to increase the team's long-term competence in performing clinical work. It is critical to recognize that in supervision, process and content are intertwined. The developing interactions between the supervisor and supervisees parallel the developing interactions between the clinical team and the family members. Accordingly, the challenges and opportunities of supervision must mirror those of treatment. Supervision can be broken down into five basic processes:

- Providing structure and consistency
- Developing skills and resources
- Promoting goal-oriented assessment and treatment planning
- Engaging the clinical team in the work
- Facilitating the ability of team members to recognize and address their own strengths and weaknesses in teamwork

These processes evolve constantly in response to the presenting needs of the clinical teams and the families with which they are working. In recognition of the need for organization and coherence, the supervisor provides a basic framework that models the structure needed to conduct the intervention. Supervision should enable the members of the clinical team to reflect on

Table 8.1. Guidelines for Supervisors

---

- Maintain focus on goals of the team's work with the family and the supervisor's work with the team.
- Avoid tangents, storytelling, and catharsis.
- Encourage use of expansion of therapeutic surface as a primary clinical technique.
- Emphasize primacy of empirical, data-based approach to promote judgment-neutral atmosphere.
- Continually address interaction between team members, including nature of collaboration and distribution of work.
- Make optimal use of each team member's skills, and offer most promising portals of strength-based intervention for family.
- Identify and ameliorate  skill deficits of team members.
- Promote bidirectional learning.
- Provide realistic but optimistic attitude.

---

their work, learn from their experiences, and acquire and implement necessary skills.

Supervision should be goal oriented, case specific, and offer opportunities for frank and open discussions that address the best interests of the clients. Finally, as with the family and the clinical team, the development of an alliance between the supervisor and the supervisees enables an effective partnership. This partnership should support ongoing, explicit assessment of the strengths and weaknesses of the teamwork.

**Responsibilities of Supervisors**

An essential responsibility of IICAPS supervisors is to provide a structure for supervision that models the structure needed to conduct the intervention. Just as the clinical team and family must develop a contract that includes mutually shared expectations and specific responsibilities, the supervisor and supervisees must establish a clear and clinically sound structure for supervision. (See Table 8.2.) In developing this structure, the partners must map out an explicit format, one that may include different elements of case presentation, goal and treatment planning, and the assessment of progress. The supervisor and supervisees must also develop a schedule of supervision that is regular and predictable, minimizes scheduling conflicts, is realistic for all parties, and minimizes time burdens for all parties. Meetings are scheduled weekly, start and end on time, and devote 15 minutes to the discussion of each case. All parties must come prepared to have a focused discussion, informed by the work of the team

Table 8.2. Responsibilities of Supervisors

- Establish clear structure with mutually shared expectations and responsibilities for both supervisor and supervisees.
- Come prepared.
- Start and end on time.
- Develop schedule of supervision that is
  - ➤ Regular, predictable, with minimal scheduling conflicts
  - ➤ Realistic for all parties
  - ➤ Minimizes time burden for all parties
- Focus on Tool preparation and creation as a means of structuring the supervision process.
- Review Tools with the clinical team in a timely fashion, since the Tools provide the cornerstone to fidelity to the IICAPS model.

with the child and family as represented by their ability to complete the Phase-appropriate IICAPS Tools together. As with therapy sessions, carefully structured supervisory sessions are not intended to promote mechanistic, repetitive discussion. Rather, the unique and challenging conditions of multiproblem families should evoke creative and dynamic dialogue between the supervisor and supervisees. Participants should view the supervisory format as a means of lending coherence to vibrant discussion, a method of focusing and operationalizing creative approaches to clinical work with children and families in need, and a venue to enhance the quality of teamwork.

### Clinical Skill Set Enhancement

The process of enhancing the skill set required of IICAPS clinicians parallels the process of Treatment Plan development. The IICAPS skill set includes:

- Mastering the use of the basic IICAPS tenets, including Principles, Concepts, and Tools
- Mastering specific skills of family therapy such as the creation of a three-generational Genogram, family timeline, and a 24-hour-day review
- Mastering individual psychodynamic and supportive psychotherapy techniques, cognitive-behavioral therapy techniques, behavioral modification skills and parent management training, crisis management, and de-escalation techniques
- Mastering intervention techniques related to intensive care management and systems change
- Mastering skills related to teamwork development and oral and written communication

## Steps of Clinical Supervision

Supervision must be flexible and individualized to the requirements of each clinician-supervisor team and each case. However, this flexibility must be contained in a structure of expected "steps" that mark the progression of information processing and planning (see Tables 8.3–5). Each of these steps may require an entire supervisory session, or several steps may occur in a single session. These suggested steps of supervision are considered an outline or a model to be kept in mind, not a rigid set of requirements to be followed mechanically.

Like the intervention itself, individual supervision can be conceived of as an iterative process with basic chronological timetables for accomplishing goals. The seven-step process encompasses a basic schedule for supervision:

Table 8.3.  Steps of Clinical Supervision for Assessment & Engagement Phase

| Step I | • Assist team to develop a concise case presentation, including: |
|---|---|
| | ➢ Demographics: child's age, ethnicity, members of immediate household |
| | ➢ Referral source |
| | ➢ Reason for referral |
| | ➢ Presenting problems |
| | ➢ History of present problems, including past treatment and medications, other relevant child, family, school histories |
| | ➢ Delineation of problems and resources in each domain |
| | ➢ Provisional DSM IV diagnoses |
| | ➢ Provisional Main Problem |
| | ➢ Provisional plan for Assessment & Engagement Phase |
| | • Assess and address any issues that require Immediate Action Plan. |
| | *(Step I should be completed by first presentation to supervisor.)* |
| Step II | • Assist team to describe family ecology by using the following devices: |
| | ➢ Generational Genogram (required) |
| | ➢ Report of 24-hour day (optional) |
| | ➢ Catalogue of family rituals, routines, and rules (optional) |
| | ➢ Assessment of child, family, school, other systems/environment (optional) |
| | ➢ Family timeline (optional) |
| | • Provisionally specify Main Problem and Strengths & Vulnerabilities in four Domains. |
| | • Construct Eco-Domain Map. |
| | *(Step II is to be accomplished in time for presentation at first rounds, three weeks after case is opened.)* |

**Table 8.4.  Steps of Clinical Supervision for Work & Action Phase**

| | |
|---|---|
| Step III | • Assist team to develop Provisional Treatment Plan with Goals and associated Action Steps and Attainment Scales.<br>• Work with team to demonstrate congruence between specific Goals, Action Steps, and Eco-Domain Map.<br>*(Step III is to be accomplished one week before the second rounds presentation, five weeks after case has been opened.)* |
| Step IV | • Conduct review of Treatment Plan signed by team and family members.<br>*(Step IV is to be accomplished every six weeks following the first rating of the Treatment Plan.)* |
| Step V | • Conduct ongoing review of progress on Treatment Plan.<br>• Review rating of Attainment Scales every six weeks or every other rounds.<br>• Assist team to revise Treatment Plan as necessary using the Treatment Refinement Process.<br>• Assist team to create draft Ending & Wrap-up Plan when Treatment Plan review and discussion with family members indicate that the Main Problem is sufficiently reduced and the goals of treatment have been achieved. |

**Table 8.5.  Steps of Clinical Supervision for Ending & Wrap-up Phase**

| | |
|---|---|
| Step VI | • Encourage co-construction of an Ending & Wrap-up Plan.<br>• Review Treatment Summary & Discharge Recommendations. |
| Step VII | • Review entire treatment experience using completed Treatment Summary & Discharge Recommendations as guidelines, to consolidate learning experiences and highlight positive intrafamilial change. |

data collection, hypothesis generation, and treatment planning and modification of the database and Treatment Plan in accordance with the results of the initial clinical intervention. There are many reasons why the supervision timeline and the completion of the Tools may be delayed. These include crises, unforeseeable session cancellations, and vacations. However, when delays occur, these issues should be discussed in supervision.

### ROUNDS: AN IICAPS FIDELITY MEASURE

Each IICAPS case must be presented in rounds every three weeks. IICAPS rounds are co-led by the IICAPS program coordinator and the IICAPS medical director and attended by all supervisors, clinicians, mental health counselors, and the IICAPS public mental health agency liaison. The timing of rounds should be as frequent and as long as needed, based upon the number of active cases being served by an individual IICAPS program. For example, an IICAPS program with a caseload of approximately 36 families would hold rounds weekly. Each rounds meeting should be scheduled for two hours to accommodate the number of cases that require presentation and discussion. Each individual case presentation at rounds is expected to take approximately 10 minutes, although, like supervisory presentations, some cases may require more time and others less.

Rounds schedules should be distributed to all attendees several days before each meeting. Rounds should complement supervision by providing input from a more "objective" audience and should inform everyone with an interest in the program about the problems and progress of each case. The rounds process promotes group learning and facilitates informed cross-coverage by clinicians and supervisors. In rounds, IICAPS clinicians are expected to provide a succinct summary of case progress since the last rounds presentation and review the goals that are expected to be achieved before the next presentation.

During rounds, attendees are expected to offer suggestions and comments to the IICAPS supervisor and the clinical team. These comments are directed toward expanding the team's knowledge of appropriate resources, psychopharmacology, relevant history, and the like. When lack of progress signals the use of the Treatment Refinement Process, the primary focus should be on the relationship between the Treatment Plan elements and the Eco-Domain Map. Does the Eco-Domain Map accurately depict the processes that sustain the Main Problem? Does each Goal and Action Step provide an achievable approach to ameliorating the processes sustaining the Main Problem as depicted by the Eco-Domain Map? The Treatment Refinement Process should occur primarily during supervision and should be used to guide the rounds discussion. Table 8.6 summarizes the timetable for rounds and the material to be presented in them.

### ROUNDS: A TIME FOR TEAM BUILDING

All members of rounds must be aware that clinician/supervisor partnership is the primary means of providing clinical direction to the team. Thus, gratuitous, affect-laden, and tangential comments are problematic. At all

Table 8.6. Timetable for Rounds and Material to Be Presented

| | | |
|---|---|---|
| *Assessment &* *Engagement Phase* | *First Rounds Presentation* (case at three weeks) | Referral source<br>Referral problem<br>Preliminary goals, and<br>  interventions<br>**Genogram**<br>**Main Problem** completed with<br>  **Severity Rating**<br>**Immediate Action Plan** completed |
| *Assessment &* *Engagement Phase* *Entering Work &* *Action Phase* | *Second Rounds Presentation* (case at six weeks) | **Genogram** completed<br>**Eco-Domain Map** completed<br>**Draft Treatment Plan** with **Main**<br>  **Problem** and **Strengths &**<br>  **Vulnerabilities** |
| *Work &* *Action Phase* | *Third Rounds Presentation* (case at nine weeks) | **Treatment Plan**, signed |
| *Work &* *Action Phase* | *Subsequent Rounds* *Presentations* | **Treatment Plan** with complete<br>**Attainment Scales** for each Goal<br>  and Action Step and dated by<br>  the team<br>IICAPS Treatment Refinement<br>  Plan (if needed) |
| *Work &* *Action Phase* | *Last Rounds of Phase* | **Ending & Wrap-Up Plan**<br>presented |
| *Ending &* *Wrap-Up Phase* | *Last Rounds* | **Ending & Wrap-up Plan** with<br>  **Attainment Scales**<br>**Treatment Summary & Discharge**<br>  **Plan** with **Attainment Scales**<br>  completed and signed by all<br>  participants |

*Note:* Items in bold should be presented as photocopies or overhead projections.

times the direction of the supervisor is paramount unless directly contravened by the medical director. The participation at rounds of a state mental health liaison to IICAPS provides an opportunity for sharing information about mental health and protective services that have a bearing on the case. When necessary, the state mental health liaison provides a channel for communication with other state mental health staff members about case-specific issues. IICAPS Services consultants attend the rounds of their assigned program sites and may offer suggestions about rounds presentation and discussion. This feedback serves primarily to illustrate the ways in which IICAPS Principles, Concepts, and Tools should be applied to rounds discussions.

The IICAPS program coordinator, with the IICAPS medical director, provides overall clinical leadership for rounds and oversees the mechanics that are crucial to their successful implementation. The coordinator's responsibilities include scheduling cases for presentation, providing a case roster with dates and times of presentation for rounds participants, having the charts on hand, keeping case presentations on time, and insuring that notes on rounds discussions are written in the chart and appropriately signed.

## IICAPS PROGRAM-SPECIFIC
## FIDELITY MECHANISMS

The Mechanisms for Fidelity at the program-specific level build upon the mechanisms for both case- and clinician-specific levels. The program-specific Mechanisms for Fidelity include initial training of all IICAPS program staff by IICAPS Services and regular program consultation by IICAPS Service consultants to each IICAPS program.

All IICAPS program staff, including mental health counselors, clinicians, program coordinators, program directors, medical directors, and supervisors, participate in a three-day, 15-hour initial training provided by IICAPS Services. The specific goals of this training are to orient all IICAPS program staff to the theoretical constructs that support the IICAPS intervention, to describe the organizational structure of the IICAPS program and network, and to present IICAPS Principles, Concepts, and Tools. The initial training, though didactic in structure, is highly interactive. Participants are encouraged to use role playing to practice the application of what they have learned to case material drawn from their own clinical experience. All participants are provided with a summary binder of the training presentation for further study and review.

Program consultation is an ongoing process led by a site consultant who is a member of the IICAPS Services staff. The site consultant serves as the primary contact between each IICAPS replication site and IICAPS Services. The overarching function of the site consultant is to support each site's adherence to IICAPS Principles, Concepts, and Tools. The responsibilities and guidelines that inform the work of each site consultant and the staff of the site are similar to those described above for the supervisor and clinical teams. The site consultant is available as needed by telephone, email, or personal visit. The site consultant assists staff members in understanding and making use of IICAPS Principles, Concepts, and Tools. The site consultant's role does not supersede the roles of the medical director, program coordinator, program director, or supervisor. Site consultants meet regularly with site-specific supervisors and medical directors to address the process of program implementation, the enhancement of supervision and rounds, and the consistent application of Principles, Concepts, and Tools to all aspects of IICAPS treatment.

## NETWORK-SPECIFIC FIDELITY STRUCTURES

The Network-specific Fidelity Mechanisms, which include IICAPS leadership and statewide quarterly plenary meetings, build on the case-specific, clinician-specific, and program-specific mechanisms. IICAPS Services produces quarterly performance reports for each program, the IICAPS Network as a whole, and the Connecticut Department of Children and Families.

Network leadership meetings are convened quarterly and are chaired by IICAPS Services staff members. The leadership meeting includes the program director, coordinator, and medical director and additional supervisors from each IICAPS program. The agenda of the meeting includes, but is not limited to, administrative issues (such as the number of open cases, number of cases on waiting list, staff changes and openings at each program, questions about financing, contract issues, and data reporting) as well as supervision and adherence issues.

A Network meeting for all Connecticut-based IICAPS teams and supervisors is held quarterly. Staffed and led by IICAPS Services personnel, these plenary meetings are open to mental health supervisors working within the state mental health agency, state mental health/IICAPS liaisons, and the state mental health administrative leadership. The agendas for Network meetings are structured to support the development of relevant clinical skills and to address salient financial, administrative, and programmatic issues.

# Chapter 9 IICAPS Development
## and Current Status

This chapter chronicles the development of IICAPS from 1996, when it began as a response to the opportunities and challenges of managed Medicaid and the perceived crisis in the children's mental health system in Connecticut, to its replication throughout the state. By 2005 IICAPS had transitioned from a single-site, innovative, but non-evidence-based practice at the Yale Child Study Center to a manualized intervention with an emerging evidence base being practiced in a 14-site statewide network. Unlike many evidence-based treatments that originate in controlled research environments, IICAPS emerged from the messy world of clinical service. Efficacy studies were not possible; measures of effectiveness needed to be put into place as soon as replication became a reality. IICAPS Services, which administers the statewide network, became the data collection arm for the network. The multiple levels of IICAPS organization were influential elements in the process of developing measures of adherence and fidelity to the model (Rogers, 1983; Woolston, 2005). The data presented here indicate a need for more scientific studies before IICAPS can claim a place as an evidence-based treatment for children with SED who are vulnerable for placement in restrictive settings.

## EVIDENCE-BASED TREATMENT
## IN AN IDEAL WORLD

Recommendations calling for the implementation of evidence-based treatment (EBT) for the care of children with SED have proliferated throughout the United States (Burns, Hoagwood, and Mrazek, 1999). Interventions with proven efficacy are those that have been subjected to the science of randomized controlled testing. Generally these interventions are delivered in academic settings to a population that is affected exclusively by the particular disorder that the intervention has been designed to treat. In addition, the providers of the treatment are seasoned clinicians who have been well schooled in the details and nuances of the intervention prior to its implementation. As a result, EBTs are empirically validated by randomized controlled trials, empirically informed by ongoing practice and empirically improved by quality assurance methods and continuous program improvement and development.

Elements that are critical to the development and replication of EBTs are mechanisms for standardizing treatment, assessing treatment effects, and managing data. The most frequently used methods for standardization of treatment are treatment manuals and adherence measures. A treatment manual is used to guide a particular intervention; if followed, it is expected to lead to the desired results for the child and/or family. It is expected that anyone providing the EBT will implement the model as instructed. Adherence to the model is the measure of how closely the manual is actually followed. There are various methodologies for the measurement of adherence, including supervision, follow-up questionnaires, and record reviews. Mechanisms for data management vary according to the design of the EBT but generally demand the submission of reporting forms and case records by clinicians, supervisors, and program administrators.

Ideally, in the development of a new EBT, basic research will have been applied to an identified clinical problem and resulted in a treatment manual to guide the implementation of the new model of care from its inception. Following implementation under ideal conditions, some of the new models will demonstrate efficacy in a controlled setting, some will demonstrate effectiveness, and some will demonstrate transportability to a real-world setting. The evolution from basic research to effectiveness in the real world requires time, money, and the ability to titrate the elements of the intervention until the most effective balance is achieved among them.

## THE HISTORY OF IICAPS:
## THE MESSY WORLD OF CLINICAL REALITY

The impetus for IICAPS has been recounted earlier in this volume. The pressing need to respond to the crisis in the children's mental health system, and the punishing effect of managed care on hospital stays and long-term treatment played important roles in the creation of the intervention. The availability of funding, coupled with clinical expertise and experience in treating children and families in home and hospital settings, provided additional motivation for the creation of the original program, the Yale Intensive In-Home Child and Adolescent Psychiatric Service (YICAPS).

In its initial phase YICAPS had the equivalent of three clinical teams, all paid for on a fee-for-service basis, with one weekly rounds for its caseload of 24 cases, the majority of which were referred from the Child Study Center's own in-patient service. YICAPS partnered with the Connecticut Department of Children and Families (DCF) in its role as the public children's mental health agency, and had a contract with one managed-care company. Within two years, YICAPS was able to obtain foundation funding for a matched controlled longitudinal observational study of dually diagnosed children referred from the in-patient unit. Although the study supported the use of home-based services as an effective treatment modality for these children, it took longer to complete than planned. However, even before there was any evidence of its effectiveness, the service was so attractive to the staff of the in-patient unit that they sought similar services from other for-profit companies. This unexpected situation reduced the number of children available for the study and delayed its completion.

In 1998 YICAPS was invited by the Department of Social Services (DSS) to be the sole provider of in-home services for children with SED who were part of a statewide network of an enhanced Medicaid program named HUSKY Plus Behavioral. Seven providers were selected to replicate the program and received some training in the model, which was still in its infancy. However, very few children qualified for the program, and the model remained virtually unused except at the original site, which had expanded to meet the demand generated by additional managed-care contracts. HUSKY Plus Behavioral ended with the advent of KidCare in Connecticut.

Within five years of its initiation YICAPS was able to expand its staff to include six teams of two persons, facilitate a second weekly rounds, and maintain an average census of 50 cases. The populations served by IICAPS have also expanded over time. The Yale site now includes IICAPS programs for medically fragile children who are at risk of hospitalization for the treatment of medical conditions such as Type II diabetes, asthma, or sickle cell disease; programs for psychiatrically impaired youth in the juvenile justice system who are at risk for placement in detention; and programs for youths returning to their homes and community from residential treatment facilities or at risk of residential treatment.

The emergence in 2003 of KidCare, a behavioral health partnership between Connecticut's DCF and DSS, provided an opportunity for additional funding and support for the YICAPS model. Renamed IICAPS, the model was selected for replication throughout the state. Clinical service providers were invited to submit proposals to replicate IICAPS as one of their clinic offerings. Fifteen sites were initially selected through this process. The rapid proliferation of IICAPS necessitated the development of a proto-treatment manual and the creation of a new entity, IICAPS Services, for the purposes of ongoing training, consultation, and network building.

### GROWING THE IICAPS NETWORK

The confluence between the state's interest in expanding its community-based programs as part of a concerted effort to reduce the number of children in hospitals and residential treatment settings and the commitment of the IICAPS developers to improved clinical practice and systems change has promoted the public/private partnership that is essential to the growth and sustainability of IICAPS. Through the processes of training, consultation, and data management for the 14 sites that now make up the network, IICAPS is able to influence the quality of practice throughout the state and to provide information to the state about the effectiveness of the intervention. The IICAPS credentialing process, a primary measure of quality assurance and fidelity, was developed with the staff members of DCF who serve as liaison to IICAPS Services. Fully implemented in the spring of 2006, the reports generated through this annual process of attending rounds, reviewing charts, and meeting with staff at each IICAPS site are used by DCF to make funding decisions concerning IICAPS providers.

The credentialing process itself places high value on the Tools that serve the multiple purposes of measuring fidelity to the IICAPS model, guiding the intervention itself and providing data for supervision. Evidence supporting the continuous and simultaneous use of the Engagement, Assessment, Treatment, and Quality-Assurance Tools is meant to assure that programs achieve recognition as authorized IICAPS sites.

Like all other IICAPS Tools, the credentialing process serves multiple aims over time. Most importantly, this process takes us a step closer to understanding if adherence to the model results in improved outcomes for children.

The Connecticut Behavioral Health Partnership now authorizes payment for IICAPS services for all Medicaid children and families who meet eligibility criteria, although few commercial insurers are willing to do so. The inclusion of IICAPS on the list of covered Medicaid services implies that these services will be funded and widely available. However, it also suggests that it will become increasingly difficult to implement randomized controlled treatment studies even though such studies are essential if the model is to achieve the status of an evidence-based treatment. A pilot study of IICAPS is currently under way at the alpha site. The study will compare service utilization, most specifically use of hospitals and other restrictive facilities, and other outcomes, of children receiving IICAPS with a group of children receiving enhanced outpatient services.

## PRELIMINARY RESULTS

During the year from January 1 to December 31, 2006, the IICAPS sites throughout Connecticut reported providing IICAPS services to a total of 660 children and youths. Table 9.1 presents demographic data for these children. Two-thirds of the children were male and one-third female. They ranged in age from 3 to 17 years at referral, with a mean of 11.1 years (standard deviation 3.31).

Children served by IICAPS are referred with a primary Axis I psychiatric diagnosis; the referral diagnoses for children whose cases were active from January 1 to December 31, 2006, are presented in Table 9.2.

Many of these children come to IICAPS services with a history of psychiatric hospitalizations. Intake data on IICAPS cases that were active from January 1 to December 31, 2006, are presented in Table 9.3.

## PRELIMINARY OUTCOME DATA

Although pilot study data are not yet available, data collected with the short form of the Ohio Youth Problem, Functioning, and Satisfaction Scales (Ohio Scales), an instrument developed to evaluate outcomes for children and adolescents receiving behavioral health services, are promising. Administered at

Table 9.1. Child Demographic Characteristics, IICAPS Active Cases, January 1–December 31, 2006

| Child demographics | IICAPS cases (N = 660) | |
|---|---|---|
| Sex[a] | | |
| Male | 414 | (62.8%) |
| Female | 245 | (37.2%) |
| Age (in years)[b] | | |
| 3–6 | 72 | (11.0%) |
| 7–9 | 129 | (19.7%) |
| 10–12 | 193 | (29.4%) |
| 13–15 | 224 | (34.1%) |
| 16 and over | 38 | (5.8%) |
| Race[c] | | |
| Caucasian | 319 | (48.7%) |
| African American | 99 | (15.1%) |
| Hispanic/Latino | 171 | (26.1%) |
| Biracial/Other | 66 | (10.1%) |

[a] Missing = 1; [b] missing = 4; [c] missing = 5.

Table 9.2. Referral Diagnoses, IICAPS Active Cases, January 1–December 31, 2006

| Referral diagnoses (Axis I disorders) | IICAPS cases (N = 660)[a] | |
|---|---|---|
| Mood disorders | 168 | (25.6%) |
| Disruptive behavior disorders | 194 | (29.5%) |
| PTSD | 53 | (8.1%) |
| Bipolar disorders | 93 | (14.2%) |
| Psychotic disorders | 32 | (4.9%) |
| Other disorders | 117 | (17.8%) |

[a] Missing = 3.

Table 9.3. Intake Data, IICAPS Active Cases, January 1–December 31, 2006

| Intake data | IICAPS cases (N = 660) | |
|---|---|---|
| Psychiatric hospitalizations (in lifetime)[a] | | |
| 0 | 279 | (42.5%) |
| 1 | 175 | (26.7%) |
| 2 or more | 202 | (30.8%) |
| Missed school during previous 60 days[a] <br> (Range = 1–60 days) | 462 | (70.4%) |
| Suspended from school in previous six months[a] | 182 | (27.7%) |
| Arrested in previous six months[a] | 58 | (8.8%) |

[a] Missing = 4.

intake and discharge to parents/guardians and youths over 12 years of age (per instrument parameters), data indicate that IICAPS is having a positive effect on the severity of children's problems, on children's functioning, on parents' and children's hopefulness, and on parents' and children's satisfaction with mental health services. These data cover IICAPS cases closed between January 1 and December 31, 2006. Findings reported in Table 9.4 are scores for those cases in which the Ohio Scales were successfully completed both at intake and at discharge (307 of 430 closed cases, or 71 percent). The number of closed cases with Ohio Scales completed by children is considerably lower because many of the children receiving services from IICAPS were too young (less than 12 years of age) to complete the youth report.

When the pilot study is completed the data will allow us to compare service utilization for children discharged from psychiatric hospital following intake to IICAPS services with service utilization by similar children receiving other community mental health services. We will also be able to compare the services used by children served by IICAPS before they entered IICAPS treatment with the services they used following treatment.

### SUMMARY

IICAPS teams are working with children with serious psychiatric disorders, over 50 percent of whom have had at least one psychiatric hospitalization as a result. These children are missing a significant number of school days;

Table 9.4. Preliminary Paired T-Test Results of Ohio Scales Scores at Discharge from Intake: Results for IICAPS Cases Closed, January 1–December 31, 2006

| Domains (discharge-intake) | N | Mean difference | Standard deviation | t-value | Pr > \|t\| | Percent change |
|---|---|---|---|---|---|---|
| Problem severity | | | | | | |
| Adult report | 307 | −10.0 | 17.3 | −10.14 | 0.0001 | −10.0 |
| Child report | 138 | −11.1 | 14.0 | −9.32 | 0.0001 | −11.1 |
| Hopefulness | | | | | | |
| Adult report | 304 | −2.3 | 5.4 | −7.38 | 0.0001 | +11.5[a] |
| Child report | 135 | −1.7 | 4.0 | −5.01 | 0.0001 | +8.5[a] |
| Satisfaction | | | | | | |
| Adult report | 304 | −2.7 | 5.2 | −9.08 | 0.0001 | +13.5[b] |
| Child report | 135 | −2.7 | 5.3 | −5.86 | 0.0001 | +13.5[b] |
| Functioning | | | | | | |
| Adult report | 305 | 6.4 | 15.6 | 7.13 | 0.0001 | +8.0 |
| Child report | 138 | 6.3 | 12.8 | 5.75 | 0.0092 | +7.9 |

[a] Negative changes in Hopefulness domain score indicate increase in Hopefulness.
[b] Negative changes in Satisfaction domain score indicate increase in Satisfaction.

many have been suspended, and others arrested. The challenges facing these children, their families, and the IICAPS teams serving them are numerous, and yet data from the Ohio Scales reveal improved child functioning and a decrease in the severity of children's problems following IICAPS. Further evaluation of outcomes of IICAPS for children and families is ongoing. Data are being collected for analyses of changes in Main Problem scores from IICAPS intake to discharge. Upon completion of the pilot study, service utilization data will allow further evaluation of the effectiveness of these services on psychiatric hospitalizations and other out-of-home placements following receipt of these services. In the meantime, analyses of Ohio Scales suggest that IICAPS has a positive impact on children with severe psychiatric disturbances, and that children and their families are satisfied with their experience of these services.

## Chapter 10  Implications for
## Public Policy

IICAPS was conceptualized as a multilevel intervention with the potential to improve the care received by individual children with serious emotional disorders and their families, to improve coordination among the systems that serve them, and to influence mental health policies and practices affecting children and youths on state and local levels. The preceding chapters have detailed the theoretical, clinical, procedural, and organizational structures that guide IICAPS interventions. On the case level, these structures are expected to lead to improved functional outcomes for the individual children with SED and families referred for IICAPS services. This chapter moves from the issues of clinical care and model specific implementation to broader issues of state and national children's mental health policies and practice standards. In particular, three areas of interest have emerged from the process of developing and disseminating IICAPS. The issues of concern relate to mechanisms for funding home-based treatment, resource development and training for clinicians providing behavioral health treatment in the home, and the process through which decisions regarding treatment options for children with SED are made. In this chapter we examine these issues and offer recommendations that may be of particular interest to mental health policy makers, public systems administrators, and child advocates.

As noted previously, the development of IICAPS was largely responsive to a crisis-driven environment that had attracted widespread governmental interest. The severity of the problems that plagued public child-serving mental health systems across the United States stimulated the formation of national and state study groups, commissions, and conferences charged with developing agendas for systems change. Compellingly, the conclusions and recommendations that have emerged from these study groups were strikingly similar (Satcher, 2000). There is a growing national consensus that the number of children requiring behavioral health intervention has outstripped the nation's capacity to serve them appropriately. The realization that providers could not adequately meet the demand for service led to the widespread view that more is needed to prevent the escalation of childhood mental health disorders. To keep the system from being immobilized by demands it could not meet, recommendations urged all those concerned about the state of children's mental health care to advance children's social and emotional health as a national priority. To achieve this goal, it was recommended that mental health systems support the promotion of early identification and treatment, actively engage families in all aspects of treatment planning, integrate services for both families and children, and implement treatments with evidence to support their effectiveness (Satcher, 2000). The IICAPS model is fully consonant with these recommendations, a central reason for its selection for replication by the public child mental health agency.

## SYSTEMS BUILDING: FUNDING

Nationally, the agenda set forth in the 2000 Report of the Surgeon General's Conference on Children's Mental Health, and enthusiastically endorsed by David Satcher, then Assistant Secretary for Health and Surgeon General of the United States, identified and supported both the promotion of mental health in children through early prevention and intervention efforts and the treatment of mental health disorders as major public health goals. Any possibility of reaching these goals in real-world settings requires the same attention to relationship building, creation of intersystemic alliances, and critical problem solving that occurs at all levels of the IICAPS model. The ability to make sustainable changes that will affect the mental health care received by American children and their families depends upon a constellation of inextricably linked factors. For example, a well-functioning mental health system must include the essential elements of comprehensive assessment, access to appropriate services, and resource availability, approachability, and acceptance. However, these components, as important as they are, are by themselves insufficient to effect the changes needed to improve our current systems. The necessary changes cannot take place without access to adequate funding for all children and families in need of care, and without the professionals and paraprofessionals with the training and supervision necessary to provide them with effective treatment.

Currently there is broad national commitment to the development and support of local mental health systems of care that draw upon the principles of CASSP (Stroul and Friedman, 1996) to inform the building of effective community collaborations. Once fully functional, these collaborations provide a mechanism to improve knowledge of and access to care, empower parents to make decisions in their child's interest, and strengthen parent-provider coalitions. However, issues of funding, not only for Medicaid-funded children but also for children who rely on commercial insurance, are seldom addressed in these venues. As IICAPS programs have proliferated, problems of insurance coverage have been revealed as barriers not only to the provision of IICAPS services but also to the broader development of effective local mental health systems of care.

An effective mental health system for children and families encompasses a continuum of care that ranges from the least to the most restrictive interventions. Costs for these services escalate in direct association with the level of restrictiveness and the intensity of the intervention. The rapid development of in-home treatment programs can be attributed, at least in part, to their widely touted potential to reduce the cost of caring for children who might otherwise be hospitalized or placed in long-term treatment facilities. When this economic argument is joined with the clinically derived presumption that children are likely to achieve maximal benefits from services that are provided in the least restrictive environments, support for in-home treatment services is further strengthened.

In Connecticut, the Department of Children and Families (DCF), a comprehensive department that serves as the designated children's mental health agency; the Court Support Services Division of the Superior Court Division for Juvenile Matters (CSSD), which operates detention and probation programs for youths in the juvenile justice system; and the Department of Social Services (DSS), the state Medicaid agency, have demonstrated a serious commitment to in-home treatment services for children with SED as an alternative to more-restrictive and more-costly residential placements. In

2000, DSS and DCF jointly commissioned a study to inform the planning for KidCare, a legislatively supported statewide initiative designed to reform Connecticut's child mental health system. The study found that the state was spending the majority of its mental health dollars on the care of a small number of children who were diagnosed with the most serious mental health problems. Specifically, 70 percent of all behavioral health dollars were being spent for psychiatric hospitalization or institutionalization of 19 percent of all children receiving Medicaid-supported mental health services. The cost of providing this level of care to an estimated 4,067 children was more than $145,000,000. At the other end of the service continuum, approximately 18,200 children were receiving community services at a cost of $61,300,000 (Connecticut Department of Social Services, 2000).

Nationally, while Medicaid expenditures for children's mental health services are expected to reach $14 billion by 2010, a similarly disproportionate amount is undoubtedly being allocated to in-patient and residential treatment. The skew toward high-end institutional services is viewed with considerable skepticism, given the increased support of mental health professionals and advocates for community-based services that adhere to CASSP principles (Pumariega, Winter, and Huffine, 2004).

The study further found that in Connecticut behavioral health services were administered by more than five state agencies plus uncounted other local agencies and schools. Given this reality, the report recommended the redistribution of existing resources, the accelerated development of community-based resources and alternatives to hospitalization and residential treatment, increased coordination at the local level, and the integration of the existing discrete funding streams (Connecticut Department of Social Services, 2000). The recommendations emanating from the study, echoed in the research literature (Burns, Hoagwood, and Mrazek, 1999; Meyers, Kaufman, and Goldman, 1999), strongly endorse the support and enhancement of accountable community-based services maintained by integrated and flexible funding sources. Although these recommendations have become a priority for both DCF and DSS, the most difficult recommendation to achieve has been the integration of funding.

In a major step towards systems change, on January 1, 2006, DCF and DSS joined together to launch the Behavioral Health Partnership (BHP), merging DSS-managed Medicaid dollars with DCF mental health treatment funds. The BHP functions as the state's payor for all covered and authorized mental health services for eligible children. The medical-necessity criteria used to manage the services covered by the BHP were established through an inclusive process spearheaded by the two state departments. An Administrative Services Organization (ASO) manages the services for the state.

Although a number of home-based services are covered by the BHP, which reimburses providers on a fee-for-service basis, IICAPS alone was selected as the first of the DCF programs previously funded under grant-based contracts to be reimbursed through a fee-for-service mechanism. Although this mechanism was seen by DCF and DSS as supportive of the expansion of IICAPS programs, the move to a fee-for-service system has been a source of concern for some providers throughout the state. Long accustomed to relying on grants and contracts for programmatic support, many providers are challenged by the transition to a competitive mental health system. Whether or not the state will achieve its goal of enabling providers to enhance capacity to meet demand is yet to be determined. The goal is well worth pursuing, and the fact that an innovative system has been implemented is promising.

Importantly, only a very few private commercial insurers have been willing to develop contractual agreements with IICAPS or other home-based providers. As a result, some poor children as well as many children of nonpoor working parents have been denied equal access to home-based, family-focused services. The reluctance of insurers to embrace in-home services as a covered service constitutes a significant barrier to the development of clinically responsive community-based mental health systems of care.

A possible strategy for addressing the failure of commercial insurers to appreciate and pay for services that play an important role in a system of care was articulated in a recent report. Among other recommendations for system improvement was a proposal to create an ongoing working group of payer, provider, advocate, patient, and agency representatives at Connecticut's Office of the Managed Care Ombudsman to ensure private insurance coverage consistent with best practices (Lieutenant Governor's Connecticut Mental Health Cabinet, 2004). A second strategy would rely upon the ability of members of the managed-care system to demand the inclusion of in-home services in the chart of covered services. Consumer pressure can be an effective tool in the process of change.

The availability of third-party funding constitutes one of the factors on which in-home and other innovative treatments depend for long-term viability. Currently providers and purchasers of care can choose from a variety of funding approaches. Contracts can be negotiated on a per-team, per-year, per-case, or per-hour basis; the last is the formula preferred by most insurers. This reimbursement strategy may also provide an unintended benefit.

A measure of program effectiveness can be derived from studying case outcomes in relation to the documented units of work performed by the team. However, a contract between a home-based treatment provider and a managed-care company stipulating the payment approach is insufficient in itself to guarantee sustainability over time. An additional and essential factor affecting the continuation and expansion of home-based treatment programs is the ability of providers to negotiate appropriate reimbursement rates that cover the cost of providing the service for the specified duration. To assure the survival as well as the effectiveness of in-home treatment models, rates must support the recommended staffing patterns. These patterns are integral to the program and reflective of the resources that are needed for the provision of intensive, closely supervised services.

A central tenet of IICAPS is that each team member makes an important contribution to the clinical work regardless of discipline. The integrated approach to treatment that characterizes IICAPS is designed to promote a true partnership between team members. This partnership is supported by IICAPS constructs, patterns of supervision, and tools. By design, it forms an important substrate that reinforces the true joining of parents and children with the team. The values of IICAPS must also be reflected at the systems level. It is essential that third-party funding support the flexibility inherent in the team partnership that is the core of IICAPS treatment.

Although master's-level clinicians function as the primary psychotherapists on the team, and take the lead in developing the psychodynamic formulations that inform the work, they have the flexibility to assume other roles. When the case dictates, master's-prepared team members may provide case management services or accompany families to appointments. At other times, the mental health counselor, who generally performs case management and advocacy functions, may move beyond those tasks to co-facilitate a family therapy session or act as a therapeutic mentor. To reinforce the flexibility that is an essential attribute of IICAPS work, programs must be reimbursed at similar rates for the time of either the master's-prepared clinician or the mental health counselor. Equalizing the rate structure for team members minimizes the possibility of model distortion and reinforces the principle of true partnership between team members. In addition, having similar rates decreases the likelihood of agency's bias toward profit maximization by overuse of a licensed professional in place of a mental health counselor. Appropriately negotiated rates should cover the full cost of care unless the program is also grant or contractually funded.

Although the most desirable rate for services is one that bundles all services at a per-hour/per-case rate, some third-party payors are reluctant to enter into such agreements, fearing they will lose control of the service mix. As insurers become more familiar with manualized, credentialed in-home service models, they may be more willing to accept fully bundled charges. In addition, the restrictive codes of the federal Health Insurance Portability and Accountability Act (HIPAA) do not support the adoption of case rates or other innovative rate-setting methodologies. For the present, it is consistent with the IICAPS model for programs to agree to dissimilar rates of reimbursement for different types of service provided by the team, independent of which team member performs the service. It is usual and acceptable for direct services, those that are provided with the child and/or his family present, to be reimbursed at a higher rate than those that are provided when they are not present. Services that do not directly include the child or family are considered indirect; indirect services may include care coordination or case management. Currently, Medicaid rules require that rates reflect whether the service being reimbursed is considered rehabilitation or case management.

In-home program administrators need to be knowledgeable about contractual and rate-setting issues. They should play active roles in contracting with funding entities and be prepared to speak to the need for adequate and appropriate reimbursement if services are to be fiscally viable. In negotiations for rates between providers and managed-care organizations, it is essential for third-party payors to understand and fiscally support the essential elements of the models they choose to offer. Unwillingness to fund all elements of IICAPS, for example, may distort the delivery of care by artificial rate splitting. If the managed-care entity is unwilling to enter into contracts that adhere to these conditions, the effectiveness of the intervention will be at stake. Under these conditions it is unlikely that a satisfactory partnership will develop. In these cases, the only remedy may be for states to develop clear policies regarding reimbursement for preferred programs that influence resistant insurers and potentially limit their ability to practice in the state.

## SYSTEMS BUILDING: TRAINING

The rapid expansion of IICAPS programs in Connecticut has not been accompanied by a parallel growth in the number of clinicians interested in or trained to provide behavioral health services for children with severe psychiatric disorders and their families in their own homes. The core competencies essential for intensive, home-based work have been well catalogued and inform the curricula of exemplary training programs. Within those institutions, the most effective approaches have been found to incorporate theory, role modeling, practice, feedback, and coaching (Osher et al., 1999). However, the principles and concepts that inform clinical practice within systems of care models do not appear to be fully integrated into the curricula of many of the behavioral health training programs that are currently graduating candidates willing to work outside a traditional outpatient setting. As a result, many job seekers are unprepared for clinical work with children with SED and unfamiliar with working in home-based settings. Given the substantial national interest in developing home- and community-based treatments, this is a poor fit.

In recognition of the problems related to professional training and resource development it is standard practice to require all IICAPS clinicians, mental health counselors, medical directors, and administrators to undergo IICAPS training before embarking on the work. Everyone affiliated with an IICAPS program is expected to participate in 15 hours of training provided by IICAPS Services training staff. Multiple training experiences have revealed some of the problems of resource development that are currently facing the field.

The manualized curriculum that guides the training consists of an introduction to IICAPS theories, Tools, Measures, and basic competencies. However, some individuals newly recruited to staff IICAPS programs lack a suitable frame of reference in which to place the information they receive. The clinical information they receive does not resonate with their work in graduate school. Their knowledge of child psychopathology and the systems that affect child functioning, the family, school, health, courts, recreation, and the like, is often sparse. In fact, few candidates for IICAPS positions are sufficiently familiar with these systems to be able to reach out and partner with them effectively.

The poor fit between the skills that unseasoned staff members bring to their work and the clinical sophistication that the treatment of children with SED and their families demands can be further exacerbated by their supervisors' lack of familiarity with the principles and theories that inform the newer system of care models. Supervisors whose careers may have matured in traditional settings in which they have acted for their clients rather than with their clients may be uncomfortable treating parents as partners in the work. Likewise, working in the child's and family's home may raise issues of safety, acceptance, or boundary setting that are not prominent factors in clinical or institutional settings. Some supervisors are unprepared for the difficult challenges of supervising teams who work in home settings in which they frequently respond to their feelings of being intimidated, anxious, or uncomfortable by becoming passive and withdrawn. Some supervisors have characterized this condition as "fading into the wallpaper."

The core competencies needed by IICAPS clinicians are multidimensional. There is no single treatment modality at the center of IICAPS interventions. IICAPS team members must be generalists, able to work with children, adolescents, and adult family members. Because the needs of each child and family must be assessed individually and in the context of their daily lives, effective training for potential IICAPS clinicians should include a level of familiarity with developmental psychopathology, adult psychopathology, marital counseling, basic knowledge of pharmacological treatments, cognitive-behavioral therapy, structural family therapy, parent management training, CASSP and Wraparound principles, and psychoanalytic theory. At this time, few training programs offer so broad a curriculum.

Recognition of the training needs at both staff and supervisory levels has prompted IICAPS Services to commit substantive resources to providing consultation to program directors and supervisors throughout the IICAPS Network. Senior IICAPS staff members facilitate monthly telephone consultations with supervisors at other IICAPS sites to address issues of supervision and adherence to the model. In addition, issues of supervising within the IICAPS model are frequently the topic of choice at the quarterly leadership meeting for all supervisors in the IICAPS Network. As home-based treatment programs gain acceptance in this country and beyond, it will be increasingly important for the theories and principles that inform them to be fully integrated into behavioral health training programs. Closer collaboration between clinical practitioners and academic training institutions should be promoted to address the challenges as well as the satisfactions of home-based child and family treatment.

## SYSTEMS BUILDING: RESOURCE DEVELOPMENT

As states have moved to expand their systems of care to include larger numbers of home-based treatment programs, they have been confronted by a shortage of qualified master's-prepared clinicians interested in careers in home-based psychiatric treatment. In response to this problem of inadequate resources, IICAPS has begun to develop policies to attract promising students to the field. IICAPS sites are encouraged to recruit and accept into mental health counselor positions individuals who have completed their bachelor's degree and have expressed some degree of interest in advanced training in the behavioral health field. Some of these individuals are uncertain about the specific discipline they would like to pursue. Others are not certain that the field is the right one for them, and want a safe way to discover the goodness of the fit between a particular career path and their talents and abilities.

As part of a clinical team, mental health counselors are presented with an opportunity to test their potential interest in pursuing a clinical discipline through firsthand exposure to real-world experience. Exposure to diverse, unfamiliar lifestyles, family practices, and complex clinical presentations is valuable preparation for a career in any area of human services. The ready availability of multiple levels of supervision and the support of professionally trained clinician co-workers are invaluable tools in the process of making career decisions. Supervisors are able to provide guidance to staff members and can assist them in making choices that are positively related to their capacity to perform in the field. In these ways, supervisors and clinician co-workers can help prepare future home-based clinicians for the challenges they will face working in programs such as IICAPS.

A second strategy for resource development supports the placement of graduate-level students in human service training programs in home-based programs. Although practice internships are commonplace for graduate schools, home-based treatment programs are less frequently selected as training venues. Policies and programs that provide state-supported internship stipends for students interested in working in home-based treatment programs would effectively increase the number of candidates prepared to enter the field upon graduation. Such policies would also promote closer collaboration between graduate schools and home-based service programs; such collaboration might bring the additional benefit of influencing curriculum development. Without well-trained personnel to staff the home- and community-based programs that are drawing widespread attention, the potential of these program models will be minimized.

## TREATMENT OPTIONS FOR CHILDREN WITH SED: POLICY IMPLICATIONS

The majority of children and adolescents referred for IICAPS services are those who have experienced chronic exposure to a broad range of environmental stressors that contribute to their psychiatric disturbances. Some of these children have suffered long-term conditions of physical or emotional neglect that have significantly damaged their self-representation; others have witnessed violence and exposure to potentially traumatic experiences that have seriously affected their sense of well-being and safety. Some of these children are known to the child welfare system, some to the juvenile justice system, and others to the child mental health system. Some children are served by all three systems. In fact, as noted earlier, the child welfare system and the juvenile justice system are frequently called upon to serve as de facto mental health systems, even though they lack the resources and expertise to respond effectively to the needs of severely troubled children. The failure of the child welfare system to address the mental health needs of children in foster care precipitated a crisis in children's mental health and stimulated a reaction that resulted in the overwhelming endorsement of the principles embodied in CASSP (Knitzer, 1982).

Treatment options for children have historically been sparse. Often the only intervention for children who were difficult to manage at home or who suffered from inadequate parenting was removal to a psychiatric hospital, residential treatment or detention center, or foster home. Placement usually meant separation from siblings and friends and resettlement in a community some distance away. Time after time, instead of improved behaviors, children often exhibited increased symptomology and eventually found themselves removed again. For most children the initial placement was likely to be followed by similar patterns of removal and placement. For example, children who enter the foster-care system in Connecticut average 3.5 placements (Martin, 1995).

Unfortunately, removal from less-than-good-enough parents and placement in foster care does not guarantee psychological or physical safety. Not only is the first out-of-home placement likely to be followed by several more; there is a real possibility that in addition to suffering the long-term consequences of the trauma of removal and loss, children will be subjected to further maltreatment. In untold instances, efforts thought to protect children from psychological distress only exacerbate the very conditions they attempt to prevent. In New Jersey, a court-approved expert assessment of the foster-care system found that one in five children in foster care is the subject of an abuse or maltreatment allegation (Kaufman and Jones, 2003). In 2005 officials in New York City canceled its contracts with an established foster-care agency because its doctored records concealed the failure of its staff to ensure that the children in the agency's foster homes received basic medical care (L. Kaufman, 2005).

Many children in institutional care do not fare much better. Recently federal investigators found "significant and wide-ranging deficiencies in patient care" at a mental health facility for children in California. Similar conditions have been cited in other states including Mississippi, Illinois and New York (Halfbinger, 2003; Bernstein, 2002).

The serious problems associated with foster and institutional care nationally provide support for clinical interventions that reduce the need to seek treatments requiring the child to live away from his family. IICAPS and other structured in-home treatments offer options that provide treatment for all family members in the service of preserving the child's ties to them. Many of these children and families test the limits of our knowledge. The paucity of developmentally appropriate permanent resources for children and youth, coupled with the high likelihood that most children will seek consciously or unconsciously to return to their families, challenges us to find pathways to engaging parents in the work of parenting. When parents are provided the treatment, guidance, understanding, acceptance, and support they need to function adequately, children can be maintained at home. As a result, their treatment issues are less likely to be compounded by the further trauma of separation and loss. For those children for whom the risk of remaining with the biologic family presents a life-threatening danger, IICAPS can be used as an intervention to promote permanency in the family in which the child is placed.

IICAPS cases have demonstrated that some families whom other providers have characterized as treatment resistant can become involved successfully in their child's treatment. The IICAPS model guides team members to break though the initial resistance by viewing the process of engaging families as the initial task of treatment. The positive alliances with family members that emerge from this process form the basis upon which the real work of stabilizing and improving child and family functioning depends. Unfortunately, many children who are removed from their homes for treatment are suffering from failures in the process to engage their families. By establishing the process of engagement as a phase of work, IICAPS has benefited a significant number of children whose parents needed attention before they could attend to their needs.

The structure of IICAPS provides multiple opportunities for each team to gain the trust, respect, and cooperation of the families with which they work. By becoming familiar with the realities of the family's life and the circumstances of their daily lives the team gathers data to inform treatment planning. By assisting children and families to identify their strengths as well as their vulnerabilities and accepting them as they are, team members take the first steps towards the development of an authentic working alliance.

The IICAPS approach is not to find fault or to assign blame. It is to discover the route by which meaningful goals can be set and progress toward the goals can be made. It is an approach to the real world of children's mental health services. IICAPS recognizes that there are precious few options for the long-term care of children and adolescents in need of adequate, consistent, and informed parents able to meet their needs. Preservation of the child's attachments to his family, culture, and history offers the best chance of stability and support for most children. However, many parents need help to provide the rules, structure, and level of parental oversight and authority that is required to meet their child's individual needs.

For this reason, IICAPS services are directed not only toward the child who is the identified patient but also to all members of his/her family. Unlike treatment provided out of the home, families must be full partners in the work. Inappropriate parental expectations that the child will be returned home fixed, often voiced when children are removed to other settings for intervention, have no place in these cases. By elevating the parent to the status of full partner, IICAPS can convert parents from passive to active participants in their child's treatment process. In some cases IICAPS teams have worked with parents to prepare them for their own long-term treatment with other community behavioral health providers; in others the work is sufficient to result in increased understanding and greater insight into their influence and importance as central players in the lives of their children. By addressing the mental health and other needs of the entire family, the IICAPS model has demonstrated its ability to assist families to remain intact. Programmatic and funding policies that support the broad dissemination and replication of IICAPS and other, similar family-focused psychiatric treatment models should reduce the number of children removed from their homes, often in failed attempts at treatment.

# References

Adnopoz, J. (2005). Working with high-risk children and families in their own homes: An integrative approach to the treatment of vulnerable children. In Lightburn, A., and Sessions, P. (Eds.), *Handbook of Community-Based Clinical Practice* (pp. 364–378). New York: Oxford University Press.

Adnopoz, J., and Culler, E. (2000). Multi-problem families: An update on intensive family preservation. Unpublished paper.

Adnopoz, J., and Ezepchick, J. (2003). Family focus: A promising strategy for serving high-risk children. In *AIA Best Practices: Lessons Learned from a Decade of Service to Children and Families Affected by HIV and Substance Abuse* (pp. 7–14). Berkeley: National Abandoned Infants Assistance Resource Center, School of Social Welfare, University of California.

Adnopoz, J., and Grigsby, R. K. (2002). High-risk children, adolescents and families: Organizing principles for mental health prevention and intervention. In Lewis, M. (Ed.), *Child and Adolescent Psychiatry: A Comprehensive Textbook* (3rd ed.) (pp. 1374–81). Baltimore: Lippincott Williams & Wilkins.

Adnopoz, J., Grigsby, R. K., and Nagler, S. (1996). Multi-problem families and high-risk children and adolescents: Causes and management. In Lewis, M. (Ed.), *Child and Adolescent Psychiatry: A Comprehensive Textbook* (2nd ed.) (pp. 1074–80). Baltimore: Lippincott Williams & Wilkins.

*AIA Best Practices: Lessons Learned from a Decade of Service to Children and Families Affected by HIV and Substance Abuse* (2003). Berkeley: National Abandoned Infants Assistance Resource Center, School of Social Welfare, University of California.

Alexander, J. F., Pugh, C., Parsons, B. V., and Sexton, T. L. (2000). Functional family therapy. In Elliott, D. S. (Ed.), *Blueprints for Violence Prevention (Book 3)* (2nd ed.).

Boulder: Center for the Study and Prevention of Violence, Institute of Behavioral Science, University of Colorado.

Behar, L. (1985). Changing patterns of state responsibility: A case study of North Carolina. *Journal of Clinical Child Psychology,* 14(3): 188–195.

———. (1986). A model for child mental health services: The North Carolina experience. *Children Today,* 15(3): 16–21.

Bernstein, N. (2002). *The Lost Children of Wilder: The Epic Struggle to Change Foster Care.* New York: Vintage.

Berrick, J., Barth, R., Needell, B., and Jonson, M. (1997). Group care and young children. *Social Service Review,* 71: 258–271.

Bickman, L. (1996). *Evaluating Managed Mental Health Services: The Fort Bragg Experiment.* New York: Plenum.

Bickman, L., Lambert, E. W., Andrade, A. R., and Penaloza, R. V. (2000). The Fort Bragg continuum of care for children and adolescents: Mental health outcomes over 5 years. *Journal of Consulting and Clinical Psychology,* 68(4): 710–716.

Blader, J. C. (2004). Symptom, family, and service predictors of children's psychiatric rehospitalization within one year of discharge. *Journal of the American Academy of Child and Adolescent Pyschiatry,* 43(4): 440–451.

Borduin, C. M., Mann, B. J., Cone, C. T., and Henggeler, S. W. (1995). Multisystemic treatment of serious juvenile offenders: Long-term prevention of criminality and violence. *Journal of Consulting and Clinical Psychology,* 63: 569–578.

Brereton, M. (2000). The Connecticut Safe Home Model: An outcome study to evaluate the effectiveness of this program for children placed in out-of-home care. Master's thesis, University of Connecticut School of Social Work.

Burns, B. J., Farmer, E. M. Z., Angold, A., and Costello, E. J. (1996). A randomized trial of case management for youths with serious emotional disturbance. *Journal of Clinical Child Psychology,* 25:476–486.

Burns, B. J., Hoagwood, K., and Mrazek, P. (1999). Effective treatment for mental disorders in children and adolescents. *Clinical Child and Family Psychology Review,* 2(4): 199–254.

Burns, B. J., Phillips, S. D., Wagner, H. R., Barth, R. P., Kolko, D. J. (2004). Mental health need and access to mental health services by youth involved with child welfare: A national survey. *Journal of the American Academy of Child and Adolescent Psychiatry,* 43(8): 960–970.

Burns, B. J., Schoenwald, S. K., Burchard, J. D., Faw, L., and Santos, A. (2000). Comprehensive community-based interventions for youth with severe emotional disorders: Multisystemic therapy and the wraparound process. *Journal of Child and Family Studies,* 9(3): 283–313.

Caspi, A., McClay, J., Moffitt, E., Mill, J., Martin, J., Craig, I., Taylor, A., Poulton, R., Campbell, Y., and Landswerk, J. (2002). Role of genotype in the cycle of violence in maltreated children. *Science,* 297: 851–854.

Caspi, A., and Moffitt, T. E. (1995). The continuity of maladaptive behavior. In Cicchetti, D., and Cohen, D. (Eds.), *Manual of Developmental Psychopathology* (Vol. 2, pp. 472–511). New York: Wiley.

Chambless, D. L., and Ollendick, T. H. (2001). Empirically supported psychological interventions: Controversies and evidence. *Annual Review of Psychology,* 52: 685–716.

Child Health and Development Institute of Connecticut. (2000). *Delivering and Financing Children's Behavioral Health Services in Connecticut.* Farmington.

Cicchetti, D., Rogosch, F. A., and Toth, S. L. (1997). Ontogenesis, depressotypic organization, and the depressive spectrum. In Luther, S. S., Burack, J., Cicchetti, D., and Weisz, J. (Eds.), *Developmental Psychopathology: Perspectives on Adjustment, Risk and Disorder* (pp. 273–313). New York: Cambridge University Press.

Cicchetti, D., and Toth, S. L. (Eds). (1999). Developmental approaches to prevention and intervention. In *Rochester Symposium on Developmental Psychopathology.* Vol. 10: *Developmental Approaches to Prevention and Intervention.* Rochester: University of Rochester Press.

Connecticut Department of Children and Families. (2003). *Guide to Connecticut Community Kidcare.* Retrieved December 30, 2005, from http://www.state.ct.us/dcf/RFP/Community_Based_Updates.htm.

Connecticut Department of Social Services. (2000). *Delivering and Financing Children's Behavioral Health Services in Connecticut (A Report to the Connecticut General Assembly, Pursuant to Public Act 99-279, Section 36).* Hartford.

D'Zurilla, T. J., and Nezu, A. M. (1999). *Problem-Solving Therapy: A Social Competence Approach to Clinical Intervention* (2nd ed.). New York : Springer.

Farmer, M. Z., Dorsey, S., and Mustillo, S. (2004). Intensive home and community interventions. *Child and Adolescent Psychiatric Clinics of North America,* 13: 857–884.

Foley, D. L., Eaves, L. J., Wormley, B., Silberg, J. L., Maes, H. H., Kuhn, J., and Riley, B. (2004). Childhood adversity, monoamine oxidase A genotype, and risk for conduct disorder. *Archives of General Psychiatry,* 61: 738–744.

Fraser, M. W., Hawkins, J. D., and Howard, M. O. (1988). *Parenting Training for Delinquency Prevention: Child and Youth Services.* New York: Haworth.

Freud, A. (1955). Safeguarding the emotional health of children. In Goldstein, J., and Katz, J. (Eds.), *The Family and the Law* (p. 1059). New York: Free Press.

Freud, A., and Burlingham, D. T. (1944). *Infants without Families: The Case for and against Residential Nurseries.* New York: International University Press.

Friedman, R., and Burns, B. (1996). The evaluation of the Fort Bragg demonstration project: An alternative interpretation of the findings. *Journal of Mental Health Administration,* 23: 128–136.

Friedman, R. M., Kutash, K., and Duchnowski, A. (1996). The population of concern: Defining the issues. In Stroul, B. (Ed.), *Children's Mental Health, Creating Systems in a Changing Society* (pp. 69–96). Baltimore: Paul H. Brookes Publishing.

Garmezy, N. (1983). Stressors in childhood. In Garmezy, N., and Rutter, M. (Eds.), *Stress, Coping, and Development in Children* (pp. 43–84). New York: McGraw-Hill.

Goldstein, J., Solnit, A. J., Goldstein, S., and Freud, A. (1996). *The Best Interests of the Child* (pp. 178–179, 252–253). New York: Free Press.

Gollwitzer, P. M. (1999). Implementation intentions: Strong effects of simple plans. *American Psychologist,* 54: 493–503.

Halfbinger, D. (2003, September 1). Care of juvenile offenders in Mississippi is faulted. *New York Times*, sec. A, p. 13.

Harlow, H. F., and Harlow, M. K. (1962). Social deprivation in monkeys. *Scientific American*, 207(5): 136.

Harrison, R. S., Boyle, S., and Farley, O. W. (1999). Evaluating the outcomes of family-based intervention for troubled children: A pretest-posttest study. *Research on Social Work Practice*, 9(6): 640–655.

Heinicke, C. M., Fineman, N. R., Ruth, G., Recchia, S. L., Guthrie, D., and Rodning, C. (1999). Relationship-based intervention with at-risk mothers: Outcome in the first year of life. *Infant Mental Health Journal*, 20(4): 349–374.

Heinicke, C. M., and Ponce, V. A. (1999). Relations-based early family intervention. In Cicchetti, D., and Toth, S. L. (Eds.), *Rochester Symposium on Developmental Psychopathology*. Vol. 10: *Developmental Approaches to Prevention and Intervention* (pp. 153–193). Rochester: University of Rochester Press.

Heneghan, A. M., Horwitz, S. M., and Leventhal, J. M. (1996). Evaluating intensive family preservation programs: A methodological review. *Journal of the American Academy of Pediatrics*, 97(4): 535–542.

Henggeler, S. W. (1999). Multisystemic therapy: An overview of clinical procedures, outcomes and policy implications. *Child Psychology and Psychiatry Review*, 4: 2–10.

Henggeler, S. W., and Borduin, C. M. (1990). *Family Therapy and Beyond: A Multisystemic Approach to Treating the Behavior Problems of Children and Adolescents*. Pacific Grove, Calif.: Brooks/Cole.

Henggeler, S. W., Pickrel, S. G., Brondino, M. J., and Crouch, J. L. (1996). Eliminating (almost) treatment dropout of substance abusing or dependent delinquents through home-based multisystemic therapy. *American Journal of Psychiatry*, 153: 427–428.

Henggeler, S. W., Rowland, M. D., Randall, J., Ward, D. M., Pickrel, S. G., Cunningham, P. B., Miller, S. L., Edwards, J., Zealberg, J. J., Hand, L. D., and Santos, A. B. (1999). Home-based multisystemic therapy as an alternative to the hospitalization of youth in psychiatric crisis: Clinical outcomes. *Journal of the American Academy of Child and Adolescent Psychiatry*, 38(11): 1331–39.

Henggeler, S. W., Schoenwald, S. K., Borduin, C. M., Rowland, M., and Cunningham, P. B. (1998). *Multisystemic Treatment of Antisocial Behavior in Children and Adolescents*. New York: Guilford Press.

Joint Commission on the Mental Health of Children. (1969). *Crisis in Child Mental Health*. New York: Harper and Row.

Kaufman, E., and Kaufman, P. N. (1992). Multiple family therapy with drug abusers. In Kaufman, E., and Kaufman, P. N. (Eds.), *Family Therapy of Drug and Alcohol Abuse* (2nd ed., pp. 72–84). New York: Gardner Press.

Kaufman, L. (2005, January 10). Foster care contracts canceled after city finds files doctored. *New York Times*, sec. B, pp. 1, 2.

Kaufman, L., and Jones, R. L. (2003, June 10). Foster care in New Jersey is called inept. *New York Times*, sec. B, p. 1.

Kazdin, A. E. (2005). *Parent Management Training: Treatment for Oppositional, Aggressive, and Antisocial Behavior in Children and Adolescents.* New York: Oxford University Press.

Kazdin, A. E., and Weisz, J. R. (1998). Identifying and developing empirically supported child and adolescent treatments. *Journal of Consulting and Clinical Psychology,* 66(1): 19–36.

Kazdin, A. E., and Whitley, M. K. (2003). Treatment of parental stress to enhance therapeutic change among children referred for aggressive and antisocial behavior. *Journal of Consulting and Clinical Psychology,* 71(3): 504–515.

Kinney, J., and Dittmar, K. (1995). Homebuilders: Helping families help themselves. In Schwartz, I. M., and Au Claire, P. (Eds.), *Home-Based Services for Troubled Children* (pp. 29–54). Lincoln: University of Nebraska Press.

Knitzer, J. (1982). *Unclaimed Children: The Failure of Public Responsibility to Children and Adolescents in Need of Mental Health Services.* Washington, D.C.: Children's Defense Fund.

Knitzer, J., and Cole, E. S. (1989). *Family Preservation Services: The Program Challenge for Child Welfare and Child Mental Health Agencies.* New York: Bank Street College of Education.

Korfmacher, J., Kitzman, H., and Olds, D. (1998). Intervention processes as predictors of outcomes in a preventive home visitation program. *Journal of Community Psychology,* 26(1): 49–64.

Lieutenant Governor's Connecticut Mental Health Cabinet. (2004). *Achieving the Promise: Recommendations of the Lieutenant Governor's Mental Health Cabinet.* Hartford.

Lindblad-Goldberg, M., Dore, M., and Stern, L. (1998). *Creating Competence from Chaos.* New York: W. W. Norton.

Lyons, J. S., and Rogers, L. (2004). The U.S. child welfare system: A de facto public behavioral health care system. *Journal of the American Academy of Child and Adolescent Psychiatry,* 43(8): 971–973.

Marsh, D. T., and Fristad, M. A. (Eds.). (2002). *Handbook of Serious Emotional Disturbance in Children and Adolescents.* New York: John Wiley and Sons.

Martin, S. (1995). Private correspondence to the author from the former deputy director, Department of Children and Families, State of Connecticut.

McCarthy, J., Meyers, J., and Jackson, V. (1999). *The Adoption and Safe Families Act: Exploring the Opportunity for Collaboration between Child Mental Health and Child Welfare Service Systems.* Washington, D.C.: National Technical Assistance Center for Children's Mental Health.

McCroskey, J., and Meezan, W. (1998). Family-centered services: Approaches and effectiveness. *The Future of Children,* 8(1): 54–71.

McGoldrick, M., Gerson, R., and Shellenberger, S. (1999). *Genograms: Assessment and Intervention.* New York: W. W. Norton.

McKay, M., and Bannon, W. (2004). Engaging families in child mental health services. *Child and Adolescent Psychiatric Clinics of North America,* 13(4): 905–921.

McKay, M., Stoewe, J., McCadam, K., and Gonzales, J. (1998). Increasing access to child mental health services for urban children and their caregivers. *Health & Social Work,* 23(1): 9–15.

Meyers, J., Kaufman, M., and Goldman, S. (1999). Promising practices: Training strategies for serving children with serious emotional disturbance and their families in a system of care. In *Systems of Care: Promising Practices in Children's Mental Health,* 1998 Series, Vol. 5. Washington, D.C.: Center for Effective Collaboration and Practice, American Institutes for Research.

Moffitt, T. E. (2005). The new look of behavioral genetics in developmental psychopathology gene-environment interplay in antisocial behaviors. *Psychological Bulletin,* 131(4): 533–554.

Nelson, D. (1988). Recognizing and realizing the potential of "family preservation." Paper presented to the Edna McConnell Clark Foundation Grantees Foundation, Washington, D.C.

Oettingen, G. (1999). Free fantasies about the future and the emergence of developmental goals. In Brandstädter, J., and Lerner, R. M. (Eds.), *Action and Self-Development: Theory and Research through the Life Span* (pp. 315–342). Thousand Oaks, Calif.: Sage.

———. (2000). Expectancy effects on behavior depend on self-regulatory thought. *Social Cognition,* 18: 101–129.

Oettingen, G., and Gollwitzer, P. M. (2001). Goal setting and goal striving. In Tesser, A., and Schwarz, N. (Eds.), *Blackwell Handbook in Social Psychology.* Vol. 1: *Intraindividual process* (pp. 329–347). Oxford: Blackwell.

Olds, D., Henderson, C., Kitzman, H., Eckenrode, J., Cole, R., and Tatelbaum, R. (1999). Prenatal and infancy home visitation by nurses: Recent findings. *The Future of Children: Home Visiting: Recent Program Evaluations,* 9(1): 44–65.

Olds, D., Hill, P., Robinson, J., Song, N., and Little, C. (2000). Update on home visiting for pregnant women and parents of young children. *Current Problems in Pediatrics,* 30(4): 107–141.

Olds, D., and Kitzman, H. (1993). Review of research on home visiting for pregnant women and parents of young children. *The Future of Children: Home Visiting,* 3(3): 53–92.

Olds, D., Robinson, J., Song, N., Little, C., and Hill, P. (1999). *Reducing Risks for Mental Disorders during the First Five Years of Life: A Review of Preventative Interventions.* Boulder: Prevention Research Center for Family and Child Health, Health Sciences Center, University of Colorado.

Osher, T., deFur, E., Nava, C., Spencer, S., and Toth-Dennis, D. (1999). New roles for families in systems of care. In *Systems of Care: Promising Practices in Children's Mental Health.* 1998 Series, Vol. 1. Washington, D.C.: Center for Effective Collaboration and Practice, American Institutes for Research.

Osofsky, J. D. (1999). The impact of violence on children. *The Future of Children: Domestic Violence and Children,* 9(3): 33–49.

Pear, R. (2003, September 1). Mental health care poor for some children in state custody. *New York Times,* p. 1.

Pires, S. (2002). *Building Systems of Care: A Primer.* Washington, D.C.: Human Service Collaborative.

President's Commission on Mental Health. (1978). *Report to the President from the President's Commission on Mental Health.* Vol. 1. Washington, D.C.: U.S. Government Printing Office.

President's New Freedom Commission on Mental Health. (2003). *Achieving the Promise: Transforming Mental Health Care in America.* Rockville, Md.

Prinz, R. J., and Miller, G. E. (1994). Family-based treatment for childhood antisocial behavior: Experimental influences on dropout and engagement. *Journal of Consulting and Clinical Psychology,* 62: 645–650.

Provence, S., Naylor, A., and Rescorla, L. A. (1983). The Yale Child Welfare Research Program: Description and results. In Zigler, E. F., and Gordon, E. W. (Eds.), *Day Care: Scientific and Social Policy Issues* (pp. 183–199). Boston: Auburn.

Pumariega, A. J., Winter, N. C., and Huffine, C. (2004). Community systems of care for children's mental health. *PSYCHLINE,* 4(3): 13–18.

Quinton, D., and Rutter, M. (1984). Parents with children in care—I. Current circumstances and parenting; II. Intergenerational continuities. *Journal of Child Psychology and Psychiatry,* 25(2): 211–250.

Rogers, E. M. (1983). *Diffusion of Innovations* (3d ed.). New York: Free Press.

Sameroff, A. J., and Fiese, B. H. (1989). Conceptual issues in prevention. In Shaeffer, D., Philips, I., and Enzer, N. B. (Eds.), *Prevention of Mental Disorders, Alcohol and Other Drug Use in Children and Adolescents* (p. 23). OSAP Prevention Monograph 2. Rockville, Md.: U.S. Department of Health and Human Services, Office for Substance Abuse Prevention.

Satcher, D. (2000). *Mental Health: A Report of the Surgeon General.* Chap. 3: Children and mental health (pp. 124–219). Washington, D.C.: U.S. Public Health Service.

Saxe, L. M., Cross, T., Silverman, N., and Doughterty, D. M. (1987). *Children's Mental Health: Problems and Services.* Durham, N.C.: Duke University Press.

Seitz, V., Rosenbaum, L. K., and Apfel, N. H. (1985). Effects of family support intervention: A ten-year follow-up. *Child Development,* 56(2): 376–391.

Snyder, W., and McCollum, E. (1999). Their home is their castle: Learning to do in-home family therapy. *Family Process,* 38(2): 229–242.

Solnit, A. (1968). In the best interests of the child and his parents. In Levitt, M., and Rubenstein, B. (Eds.), *Orthopsychiatry and the Law* (pp. 114–126). Detroit: Wayne State University Press.

———. (1976). Marriage: Changing structure and functions of the family. In Vaughn, V. C., and Brazelton, T. B. (Eds.), *The Family--Can It Be Saved?* (p. 234). Chicago: Year Book Medical Publishers.

———. (1980). Too much reporting, too little service: Roots and prevention of child abuse. In Gerbner, G., Ross, C., and Zigler, E. (Eds.), *Child Abuse: An Agenda for Action* (pp. 135–146). New York: Oxford University Press.

Solnit, A., Adnopoz, J., and Fallon, T. (1993). Evaluation of the Mental Health Services Program for Youth. In Saxe, L., *Interim Report to the Robert Wood Johnson Foundation.* Waltham, Mass.: Brandeis University.

Solnit, A., Adnopoz, J., Saxe, L., Gardner, J., and Fallon, T. (1997). Evaluating systems of care for children: Utility of the clinical case conference. *American Journal of Orthopsychiatry,* 67(4): 554–567.

State of Connecticut. (2000). *Report of the Governor's Blue Ribbon Commission on Mental Health.* Hartford.

Stroul, B. A., and Friedman, R. M. (1985). *A System of Care for Severely Emotionally Disturbed Children and Youth* (Rev. ed.). Washington, D.C.: Georgetown University Child Development Center, National Technical Assistance Center for Children's Mental Health.

———. (1996). The system of care concept and philosophy. In Stroul, B. (Ed.), *Children's Mental Health: Creating Systems of Care in a Changing Society* (pp. 3–22). Baltimore: Paul H. Brookes Publishing.

Stroul, B. A., Pires, S. A., Armstrong, M. I., and Zaro, S. (2002). The impact of managed care on systems of care that serve children with serious emotional disturbances and their families. *Children's Services,* 5(1): 21–36.

Tebes, J., Kaufman, J., Adnopoz, J., and Racusin, G. (1999). Reducing risk for children of parents with serious mental disorders through family support. *Yale Psychiatry,* 8(1): 6.

Von Bertalanffy, L. (1968). *General System Theory.* New York: George Braziller.

Weersing, V. R., and Weisz, J. R. (2002). Mechanisms of action in youth psychotherapy. *Journal of Child Psychology and Psychiatry,* 43(1): 3–29.

Weisz, J. R., Huey, S. M., and Weersing, V. R. (1998). Psychotherapy outcome research with children and adolescents: The state of the art. In Ollendick, T. H., and Prinz, R. J. (Eds.), *Advances in Clinical Child Psychology* (Vol. 20, pp. 49–92). New York: Plenum.

Weisz, J. R., Weiss, B., Han, S. S., Granger, D. A., and Morton, T. (1995). Effects of psychotherapy with children and adolescents revisited: A meta-analysis of treatment outcome studies. *Psychological Bulletin,* 117: 450–468.

Wells, K. (1995). Family preservation services in context: Origins, practices and current issues. In Schwartz, I. M., and Au Claire, P. (Eds.), *Home-Based Services for Troubled Children* (pp. 1–28). Lincoln: University of Nebraska Press.

Wells, K., and Tracy, E. (1996). Reorienting intensive family preservation services in relation to public child welfare practice. *Child Welfare,* 75(6): 667–692.

Woodford, M. (1999). Home-based family therapy: Theory and process from "friendly visitors" to multisystemic therapy. *Family Journal: Counseling and Therapy for Couples and Families,* 7(3): 265–269.

Woolston, J. L. (1988). Theoretical considerations of the adjustment disorders. *Journal of the American Academy of Child and Adolescent Psychiatry,* 27: 280–287.

———. (1989). Transactional risk model for short and intermediate term psychiatric inpatient treatment. *Journal of the American Academy of Child and Adolescent Psychiatry,* 28: 38–41.

———. (2005). Implementing evidence-based treatments in organizations. *Journal of the American Academy of Child and Adolescent Psychiatry,* 44: 1313–1616.

Woolston, J., Berkowitz, S., Schaefer, M., and Adnopoz, J. (1998). Intensive, integrated, in-home psychiatric services: The catalyst to enhancing outpatient intervention. *Child and Adolescent Psychiatric Clinics of North America,* 7(2): 615–633.

# Index

The letter *t* following a page number denotes a table; the letter *f* denotes a figure.